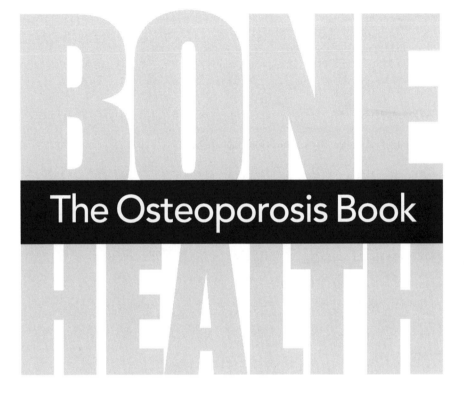

# The Osteoporosis Book

**GWEN ELLERT** RN, MEd
**ALAN LOW** PharmD, CCD
**JOHN WADE** MD, FRCPC

osteoporosisbook.com

Trelle Enterprises Inc.

**Library and Archives Canada Cataloguing in Publication**
Ellert, Gwen
　　　The osteoporosis book : bone health / Gwen Ellert, Alan Low, John Wade. – 3rd ed.

ISBN 978-0-9692210-3-6
　　　1. Osteoporosis–Popular works. 2. Osteoporosis–Prevention.
3. Osteoporosis–Treatment. I. Low, Alan, 1968- II. Wade, John
III. Title.
RC931.O73E44 2011　　　　616.7'16　　　　C2010-907821-7

**Published in Canada by**
Trelle Enterprises Inc.
Vancouver, BC
Tel 604-874-6197
www.osteoporosisbook.com

First Edition – September 1993
Second Edition – May 2001
Third Edition – May 2011

**NOTICE**
This text is not intended as a substitute for personal medical advice. Before taking any form
of treatment, you should always consult with your physician.

Illustrations by Dave Hancock
Edited by Bruce Wells
Design by Leap Creative Group, Inc.
Printed in Canada by Hignell Printing, Winnipeg, Manitoba

osteoporosisbook.com

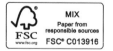

MIX
Paper from
responsible sources
FSC
www.fsc.org　FSC® C013916

# BONE

The authors wish to thank Brian C. Lentle, MD, FRCPC, FRCR, FACR for sharing his expertise and for his kind contribution to the third edition of The Osteoporosis Book.

# HEALTH

# Contents

*Foreword by Jonathan D. Adachi MD, FRCPC*                                    9

**INTRODUCTION**

    Caring About Your Bone Health                              11

**PART ONE: THE BASICS FOR MEN AND WOMEN**

1.  What is Happening on the Inside?                              16
      *Bone Growth and Development*
      *Inside the Bones*
      *Primary and Secondary Osteoporosis*

2.  Menopause and Hormone Therapies                          34
      *Menopause*
      *Hormone Therapies*

3.  Testosterone, Andropause and Bone Loss                   44
      *Calling All Men*
      *Testosterone Levels*
      *Testosterone Replacement Therapy*
      *Other Treatments for Osteoporosis in Men*
      *Monitor Your Therapy*

**PART TWO: OSTEOPOROSIS PREVENTION**

4.  Calcium                                                  54
      *Diet and Bone Health*
      *Calcium*
      *Calcium Intake*
      *Calcium Supplements*

5.  Vitamin D and Other Vitamins and Minerals          73
    *Vitamin D*
    *Vitamin D Sources*
    *How much Vitamin D do I need?*
    *Other Vitamins and Minerals*
    *Alkaline (Basic) or Acid-Producing Foods and Bone Health*

6.  The Importance of Exercising and Safe Movement      83
    *Non Weight-bearing Activities*
    *Weight-bearing Activities*
    *Walk, Walk, Walk*
    *Joining a Fitness Program*
    *Exercise Considerations*

7.  Exercises                                            90
    *Choosing the Appropriate Exercises*
    *Charting Your Course*
    *Set A: Stretching Exercises*
    *Set B: Balance Exercises*

## PART THREE: CLINICAL EVALUATIONS AND TREATMENTS

8.  Clinical Evaluation to Assess Bone Health           132
    *Risk Factors for Osteoporosis*
    *Risk Factors for Fall and Fracture*
    *Ways to Assess Your Bone Health*

9.  10-Year Fracture Risk Assessment Tools             145
    *Assessing Your Fracture Risk*
    *FRAX*
    *CAROC Fracture Risk Assessment*

10. Fall and Fracture Prevention and Post-Fracture Care  152
    *Fall Prevention*
    *Fracture Prevention*
    *Post-Fracture Care*

11. Medical Treatments     165
   *Mechanism of Action*
   *Route of Administration*
   *Benefit, Risk and Cost Factors*
   *Side Effects and Rare Events*
   *Treatments for Osteoporosis*
   *Cancer Medications and Glucocorticoids:*
      *Treatments to Protect Bone*
   *Future Drug Therapies*

12. Understanding Health Headlines     193
   *Be Cautious When Reading Headlines*
   *Research Terminology*

**PART FOUR: TAKING CONTROL OF YOUR BONE HEALTH**

13. Bringing It All Together     202
   *Managing the Prevention of Bone Loss*
   *Managing Your Osteoporosis*

14. Living Well with Osteoporosis     212
   *Daily Movement and Activities*
   *Daily Living Tasks*
   *Managing Pain*

15. Examples of Patients with Osteoporosis     226

16. Resources     236

17. Glossary     242

   *Bone Health Care Plan*     251

   *Acronyms and Abbreviations*     252

   *Acknowledgements*     254

   *About the Authors*     256

# Foreword

The field of osteoporosis is changing with increased attention being paid to the importance of vitamin D, fracture prevention and the development of new tools to identify those at risk of fracturing.

The third edition of *The Osteoporosis Book* refocuses us from disease treatment to fracture prevention. Fracture risk assessment tools like FRAX and CAROC are discussed to help you to understand the risk factors that might affect your bone health and your risk of fracturing.

Several chapters show you how to manage your bone health and include updated information on calcium, vitamin D and exercise. Vitamin D has been a topic of much attention and is well reviewed. This is discussed with helpful tips on how you might increase your intake and exposure to vitamin D. Sources of calcium and other minerals are also discussed. The exercise chapter is well illustrated with exercises that you can do. This is extremely important for people who want to take charge of their condition. Various new and old treatment options are discussed, with very recent therapies being included and new information of old therapies being shared with you. Risks and benefits of these treatment options are discussed to help you and your physician determine the treatment that is right for you. Information about non-pharmaceutical options, such as vertebroplasty and kyphoplasty, are also presented.

People who suffer from chronic disease like osteoporosis benefit from knowledge about their disease. This book is well written and will provide the level of knowledge that will be helpful to all who are interested in osteoporosis. I believe that this book will be of particular interest to people who suffer from osteoporosis, their relatives, and the healthcare professionals who care for them.

**Jonathan D. Adachi MD, FRCPC**
*Professor, Department of Medicine, McMaster University*
*Member, Board of Directors and Council of Scientific Advisors,*
*International Osteoporosis Foundation*

# Caring About Your Bone Health

We've all seen the headlines: "New drug reduces fractures by 70 percent." Wow, I need to tell my doctor to put me on that drug. Or "Calcium pills raise heart risk." I know I need to take calcium to maintain strong bones, but is it worth the risk if taking calcium pills leads to heart problems?

We've also seen the many advertisements on television about how this drug or that drug can help us address a health problem or make us feel better. They tell us all about the potential side effects and advise us to "be sure to talk to your doctor before taking any medication." Sound advice.

How about the times we have stood in the aisle of a drug store looking at the shelves of vitamins and minerals with their various levels of dosing and wondering which ones to choose? 400IU, 1,000IU or 5,000IU? Are they all the same or is a name brand different than a generic brand?

Of course we can ask our doctor or the pharmacist for advice, or search the internet for information and we should take advantage of these opportunities. At the end of the day however, decisions about the vitamins or medications we take or headlines we believe are ours to make.

This book is about helping you to understand how your bones work, how to prevent bone loss and fractures and how your bones are affected when you have osteoporosis. It is about helping you to know what is going on inside your body so you can ask the right questions and get the information you need in order to make relevant and timely decisions about your own health. This book will help you to better understand the issues so you become better informed and ask the important questions when you seek professional advice.

In the chapters ahead, we are going to review the various risk factors for osteoporosis and falls and fractures. We will introduce you to methods for self-managing your bone health and preventing falls and fractures. We're going to discuss the different treatment options for both women and men who have osteoporosis. You will discover exercises that can help you to feel better and to reduce your risk of fractures so you can maintain the lifestyle you choose while living with osteoporosis.

The first two editions of *The Osteoporosis Book* provided readers with basic information about bone health and offered tips for maintaining a healthy lifestyle while living with osteoporosis. In the third edition, we expand upon that information and include more information about prevention, self-management, individualizing your care plan and post-fracture care.

In this edition, we include more technical terms and explain some science in more detail. With easy access to fracture assessment tools, we encourage you to do your own bone assessment to gain an understanding of what affects your bone health. It may be important that you discuss your assessment with your doctor. Also, it is important that you know how to decrease your risk of fracture and to manage post-fracture care.

We include information to help you understand media headlines and some research terms. Examples of patients with osteoporosis help to illustrate different situations. To support and encourage patient-centered care, we have expanded the list of resources you can use and provided a more detailed glossary so you can become familiar with the language that is used to discuss your bone health.

Although awareness of bone health and osteoporosis is improving, perspective is often missing. This edition of *The Osteoporosis Book* offers that perspective. We know we need calcium, vitamin D and weight-bearing exercise to decrease our risk of falling and fractures. However, we still stare at the store shelf wondering, "Do I need a calcium pill?" "If I have milk on my cereal and in my coffee, is that enough calcium for the day?" "Does it really matter what calcium or vitamin D I buy and what time of day I take the pill?"

Or we will stand at the door looking at the gym equipment knowing that movement is necessary to keep our bones strong but, "Does it really matter what exercises I am doing as long as I am moving?" "How do I manage with my heart and joint issues and still lift weights?" We wonder at what point the idea of taking medication goes from "it might help" to "it is recommended."

Some believe this is all fear mongering from the doctors and drug companies to make us think that something as natural as aging and bone loss requires yet another drug? The good news is that this belief makes us wisely question our healthcare and look for credible evidence-based information and resources. *The Osteoporosis Book* will guide you from prevention to treatment to post-fracture care. We will help you find answers to questions about your bones. Questions such as, "Am I really at risk of breaking a hip or fracturing my spine?" "How likely is it that I will end up losing my ability to be independent and live where I choose?" "How can I best maintain or improve my bones?"

Osteoporosis is a major health and economic problem and is increasingly common with age in both men and women. Today's healthcare systems are moving towards patient-centered care. The goal of this type of care is to encourage patient empowerment through education and support from the healthcare team. It requires you to take responsibility for your health and the care you need, to educate yourself about your body, how it works and what issues are important to your health and well-being. The more you know and understand, the more confident you will be in participating in your own care and posing the right questions to your healthcare team.

A speaker at a medical conference recently told his colleagues, "If we don't ask the patient, they will not tell us." As a patient, it is your responsibility to tell the doctor what you want him or her to know. Speak up, ask questions, seek clarification and share your thoughts and opinions. Do not wait to be asked.

We have the right and responsibility to question, clarify and understand treatments that are being suggested. Often, there are many options to choose from. Your doctor will discuss the risks and benefits of a treatment, given your health situation. However, the choice of treatment is yours to make and follow. This holistic, patient-centered care approach is designed to encourage and support the education and empowerment of patients as they become an important part of their healthcare team.

It's your life. Participate in it. Be active and attentive. Be involved so the care and treatments you receive are individualized to your needs and preferences. If you have osteoporosis, don't waste time worrying about it, being ill or less well than you can be. Find the answers you need. Seek out information until you are satisfied that you understand the issues and how they relate to your situation. Focus on what you can do rather than on what you cannot do.

## Introduction Key Points*

- **Empowerment supported by good information is key to the prevention and treatment of osteoporosis and fracture.**

- **Appropriate patient-centered care will help you to succeed in achieving your individualized goals.**

*Key points at the end of each chapter provide a summary of that chapter. You may wish to review the key points first to help in guiding you through the chapter.*

# PART ONE

# The Basics for Men and Women

**What is Happening on the Inside**

**Menopause and Hormone Therapies**

**Testosterone, Andropause and Bone Loss**

# What is Happening on the Inside

**The goal is to prevent osteoporosis and fractures. There are things you can do to reduce bone loss and prevent falls or decrease the risk of fracture from a fall.**

---

Bone is a living tissue that is continually formed (being made) and resorbed (removed) over a seven-year cycle. This is called bone remodeling. The adult human skeleton consists of 206 bones. These bones provide a rigid structure that supports and protects the internal organs. They are also a point of attachment for muscles and tendons to facilitate body movement.

The connection between two or more parts of the skeleton is called a joint. Joints enable the body to be flexible and to rotate. The body's movement also depends on muscle action. For movement to occur, one or two main muscles contract while many other supporting muscles simultaneously contract or relax.

To move easily, your body must have bones that are strong enough to support your body weight, joints that are flexible enough to allow movement, and muscles that are healthy enough to contract and relax. This contracting and relaxing of the muscles causes a bend at the joint that enables the body to move. If any of the bone, muscle or joint groups are not healthy, movement may be difficult and you may be at risk of a fall and fracturing a bone.

## BONE GROWTH AND DEVELOPMENT

Bone density and strength occurs through remodeling. Bone tissue continually renews itself by remodeling – a process whereby small pits or tiny holes are created by osteoclast (removal) cells. These holes are then filled with new bone by osteoblast (building) cells. At any one time, less than one percent of the bone is involved.

Bone remodeling goes through various stages. It starts with the resting stage and the cells communicating with each other. The osteocyte cells deep within the bone signal when the bone needs to build up or break down. This signal triggers this bone remodeling. The bone resorption (removal) stage occurs when the osteoclast cells are activated. Over the next two to four weeks, the osteoclast cells remove old or damaged bone, leaving new pits or tiny holes where the old or damaged bone has been removed. This next stage occurs when pre-osteoblast cells are recruited and the tiny holes are cleaned and prepared for formation of new bone. For the next one to five months, the osteoblast cells build new bone by filling up these small pits and cracks. The new bone forms in the holes and hardens as calcium is deposited. This is called the formation stage. The hardening or mineralization completes the bone remodeling process until the next time it starts.

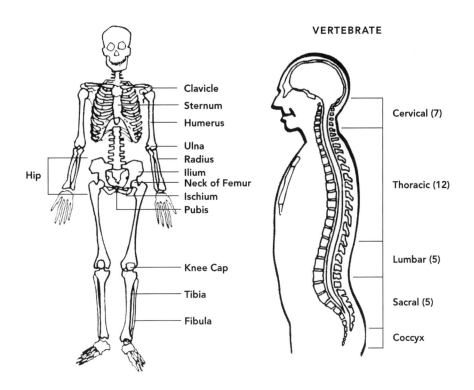

VERTEBRATE

Clavicle
Sternum
Humerus
Ulna
Radius
Ilium
Neck of Femur
Ischium
Pubis
Hip
Knee Cap
Tibia
Fibula

Cervical (7)
Thoracic (12)
Lumbar (5)
Sacral (5)
Coccyx

The diagram on this page shows how the remodeling stages develop and maintain bone by removing old bone and forming new bone. Bone mass is determined through this cycle of removal and formation. Essentially, if the same amount of bone is removed as is formed, the bone stays the same. If more bone is removed than is formed, the bone loses its mass. As bones grow, they generally become stronger.

The osteocytes, osteoclasts and osteoblasts are regulated, in part, through a protein called RANK Ligand (RANKL). This protein stimulates cells that grow to become osteoclast cells, which remove bone. The more the osteoclast cells are activated, the more bone is removed. Because the body does not want too much bone removed at one time, it produces a protein called osteoprotegerin (OPG). This protein slows down bone loss and helps to maintain a balance between bone resorption and

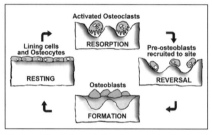

Stages of Bone Remodeling

formation. However, remember as we age the body will naturally remove more bone than is formed. Osteoporosis can occur when the quantity and quality of the bone decreases to the point where there is a significant risk of fracture. Later in the book we will discuss how drug therapy works to either slow down the bone removal cells (anti-resorptive drugs) or increase the bone building cells (anabolic drugs) in order to decrease bone loss.

Scientific knowledge of the cells and signals relating to bone resorption and formation is constantly improving. Past research concentrated on the influence of environmental factors, such as nutrition and lifestyle and their impact on osteoporotic fractures. We now understand that bone formation is influenced by general health, exercise and diet. A proper supply of minerals, such as calcium and vitamin D, is important.

When bone starts to form in the unborn child, the major portion of the skeleton is made up of cartilage – a dense connective tissue that is progressively replaced by calcified true bone. Throughout childhood, particularly during the rapid growth of adolescence, bone is formed at a greater rate than it is resorbed. As the body grows, bone generally becomes longer, denser and stronger. Exercise and a diet rich in calcium and vitamin D are necessary to ensure optimal bone growth and strong bones for the future.

By the time most people reach the age of 20, their bones have stopped growing longer. However, bone density can continue to increase until the mid-thirties, at which time bone density reaches its maximum. This maximum is called peak bone mass (PBM).

Age and gender affect bone growth, and not all bones grow at the same rate. In women, for example, PBM of the lumbar (lower) spine can be achieved in the late thirties, while PBM in the hips can be achieved in the teen years. In men, PBM of the lumbar spine is reached in the late twenties and in the hip up to the mid-thirties.

Once peak bone mass is reached, bone formation no longer keeps up with bone removal. From about age 40, the balance starts to shift. A little more bone is resorbed than formed and the bones may start to weaken.

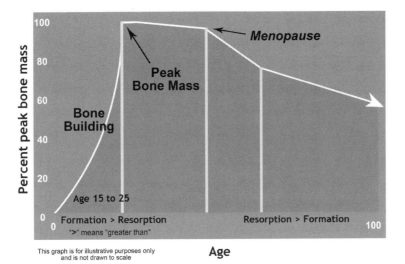

**Menopausal Effects of Bone**

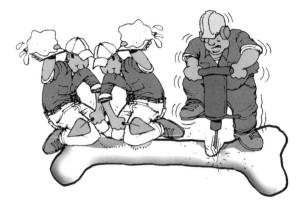

Throughout childhood, bone is formed at a greater rate than it is resorbed.

Around age 30 to 40, bone formation and resorption is close to balanced.

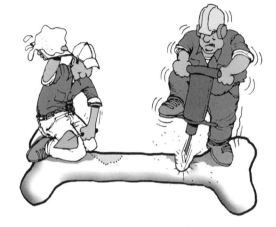

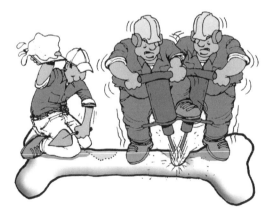

By about age 40, the balance has shifted and more bone is resorbed than formed.

Age-related bone loss occurs at a rate of about half a percent to one percent per year. The rate of bone loss increases significantly in women during peri-menopause and after menopause. For the first five or six years following menopause, a woman can lose two to five percent of her bone density each year. This increase in post-menopausal bone loss is primarily caused by a drop in estrogen production. By age 65 or 70, bone loss in women slows and the rate of bone loss is similar in men and women. More on menopause, increased fracture risk and preventative measures will be discussed in the next chapter.

## INSIDE THE BONES

A bone under stress (when the bone structure is not strong or the bone density is low) is at risk of fracture. The degree of risk depends on the bone's strength and the amount and direction of stress placed on it.

Because more bone is resorbed than formed after we reach our late twenties to mid-thirties, the density of our bones declines as we age causing bones to become weaker. For an older person with low bone density, the amount of stress required to cause a fracture will be much less than for a younger, healthy person. A small fall or an even unexpected twist could result in a fracture.

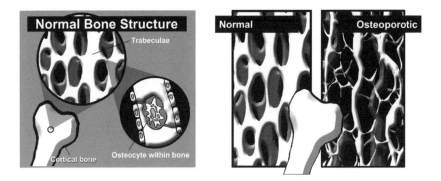

The human body has two types of bone: cortical and trabecular. Cortical bone is compact, dense bone that forms the outer shell of all bones. Trabecular bone is a less dense bone surrounded by the harder cortical bone. Bones that make up the spine are largely composed of trabecular bone. Consequently, the spine is often the first part of the body to show signs of osteoporosis and is most vulnerable to fractures. The other most common body parts to fracture are the hip, wrist, humerus (upper arm bone) and ribs.

Bone loss in the spine may cause the vertebrae to become weak and porous. If this loss continues, the vertebrae may become so thin that they eventually collapse under the weight of the body, perhaps during a simple, everyday movement.

In very severe and advanced stages of osteoporosis, more than one vertebra may collapse. Vertebrae can collapse all at once or they may collapse over a period of time. Collapsed vertebrae will cause the rib cage to tilt downward and rest on the hip bone or pelvis. The internal organs are forced outward, resulting in a protruding abdomen or stomach. More than half of vertebral fractures do not result in pain, but if pain does occur, it may be persistent pain.

Collapsed vertebrae will result in a person becoming shorter. You may see an increase in the outward curve in the upper spine (kyphosis or spinal curve) and an inward curve in the lower spine (lordosis) or a flat back. Vertebral fractures may result in serious concerns regarding image, independence and self-esteem. We discuss ways of managing these concerns later in the book.

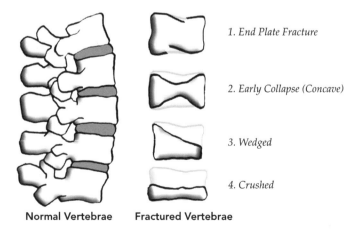

1. *End Plate Fracture*

2. *Early Collapse (Concave)*

3. *Wedged*

4. *Crushed*

**Normal Vertebrae**     **Fractured Vertebrae**

The most physically significant body part for a fracture is the hip. Hip fractures can occur as a result of a fall, but in many cases there may be no apparent cause. Hip fractures have a great potential to be disabling and life threatening.

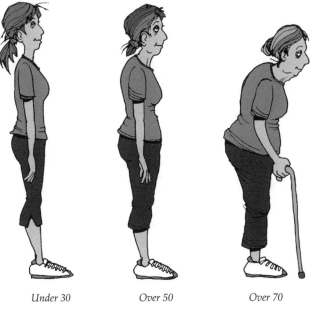

*Under 30*  *Over 50*  *Over 70*

**Collapsing vertebrae leading to a curved spine (kyphosis)**

## Nutrients, Hormones and Bone

Certain nutrients need to be properly absorbed in order to help maintain bone. These nutrients, such as calcium, phosphorus and some vitamin D, come from our diet. Our bodies break down and digest the food we eat. The foods that cannot be digested are passed out of our bodies. Digested foods release nutrients that are absorbed into the bloodstream, mainly from the small intestine.

The bloodstream carries the absorbed nutrients through the body. The tissues take the nutrients they need from the blood. However, the body must have a way of telling whether the blood has the right amount of nutrients. Any condition that affects the absorption of these nutrients may affect the bones. Detecting the amount of nutrients available is the role of certain hormone producing glands.

Hormones involved in regulating blood calcium (essential for bone health) are:

- *Parathyroid secreted by the parathyroid gland*

- *Calcitonin from the thyroid gland*

- *Calcitriol produced from vitamin D converted in the liver and in the kidney*

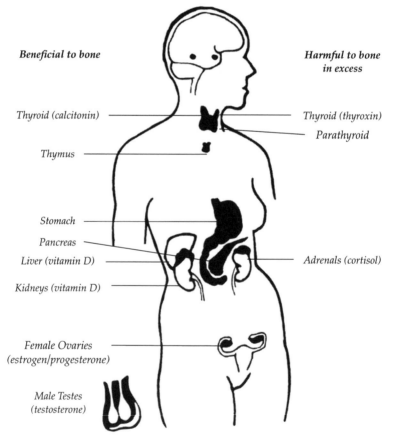

*Beneficial to bone*

*Harmful to bone in excess*

*Thyroid (calcitonin)*

*Thyroid (thyroxin)*

*Parathyroid*

*Thymus*

*Stomach*

*Pancreas*

*Liver (vitamin D)*

*Adrenals (cortisol)*

*Kidneys (vitamin D)*

*Female Ovaries (estrogen/progesterone)*

*Male Testes (testosterone)*

**Glands and Hormones**

Other hormones that affect bone are:

- *Thyroxine from the thyroid gland*

- *Insulin from the pancreas*

- *Growth hormone from the anterior pituitary gland*

- *Cortisol from the adrenal glands*

- *Estrogen and progesterone from the ovaries in women and fat tissue*

- *Testosterone from the testes in men*

Any condition that affects these glands may affect the bones. Changes in the normal levels of hormones may cause an imbalance in bone formation and resorption. An imbalance may result in more bone being taken away than is formed, causing weak bones. If you have any problems with your glandular (endocrine) system, discuss your bone health with your doctor or a specialist in bone disease. If the problem is hormone related, your doctor may refer you to an endocrinologist.

## Genetics and Lifestyle

Genetics and lifestyle have significant influences on our bone health. Research into genetic factors that contribute to osteoporosis suggests that genetic markers may identify some individuals who are at risk of developing osteoporosis. Testing people when they are young and identifying those who are at high risk of osteoporosis may necessitate lifestyle changes, including taking medications to decrease the risk. However, proper genetic testing is expensive and inconclusive as to what actions will give the best outcome.

We should all concentrate on reaching our best peak bone mass, maintaining the bone we have and living a bone healthy lifestyle. If you fracture a bone, talk to your doctor about osteoporosis. The following chapters in this book will help you identify issues and topics to discuss with your doctor or healthcare provider.

## PRIMARY AND SECONDARY OSTEOPOROSIS

- *Primary osteoporosis is when there is no obvious cause of bone loss other than genetically-related and/or age-related changes.*

- *Secondary osteoporosis is when disease conditions, immobility or medication are identified as the cause of the bone loss or a fracture.*

The amount of calcium in the bone can be identified through a bone mineral density test. This test is used to diagnose osteoporosis in post-menopausal women and older men. Osteoporosis can also be diagnosed if you have a low-trauma fracture (for example, caused by a fall from a standing height or less). Some experts refer to a fracture as a "bone attack" to impress upon people the magnitude of the problem.

To determine if low bone density is due to primary osteoporosis or another condition that may be causing bone loss, your doctor or other healthcare provider may use the following blood tests (refer to the glossary for more details):

- *Complete blood count (CBC)*

- *Serum calcium*

- *Serum creatinine and calculated creatinine clearance*

- *Alkaline phosphatase*

- *Thyroid-stimulating hormone (TSH)*

Additional tests that may be necessary after a clinical evaluation include:

- *Blood tests for celiac disease*

- *Serum Parathyroid hormone (PTH)*

- *Serum 25-hydroxy vitamin D*

- *Serum immunoelectrophoresis*

- *24-hour urine: calcium and cortisol*

- *Sex hormones: Estradiol; Follicle Stimulating Hormone (FSH); Luteinizing Hormone (LH); Testosterone (in men – total, as well as free or bound); Sex Hormone Binding Globulin (SHBG) (in men and women)*

# Primary Osteoporosis

## POST-MENOPAUSAL OSTEOPOROSIS IN WOMEN

Bone loss is believed to be a result of a natural decrease in estrogen associated with menopause. Rapid bone loss at a rate of two to five percent a year occurs for the first five or six years of menopause. Five or six years after menopause, the rate of bone loss gradually slows to one percent per year. Women can lose as much as 20 percent of their bone mass during this period. Women at the highest risk of developing osteoporosis are individuals who achieved only a low peak bone mass by the time they reached their thirties. Not all women develop post-menopausal osteoporosis, but menopause is considered a risk factor for osteoporosis.

Factors that affect the development of post-menopausal osteoporosis include genetic predisposition (an example might be a close family member fractured a hip due to osteoporosis), peak bone density levels, and diet and exercise over a person's lifetime (the importance of diet and exercise are discussed later in this book). It is important to understand that diet and exercise may not be sufficient in and of themselves to prevent bone loss in early post-menopausal women. Genetics, lifestyle and medical conditions also play a role.

Menopause before the age of 45 is a risk factor for low bone density. That's because women who go through menopause early experience the loss of estrogen earlier in life than women who reach menopause at a later age.

## AGE-RELATED OSTEOPOROSIS IN MEN AND WOMEN

Bone loss may start at a rate of half to one percent a year after a person reaches his or her late twenties or mid-thirties. Peak bone density levels, which are partially determined genetically, will have an effect on the development of osteoporosis. The rate of bone loss can accelerate in extreme old age due to immobility.

As men and women age, they may need to make lifestyle changes to reduce bone loss. This can include increasing weight-bearing and balance exercises, and changing to a diet rich in calcium and sufficient vitamin D. Generally, 1,000mg to 1,200mg of elemental calcium (amount combined from supplements and diet) and vitamin D 800IU to 2000IU (international units) daily are recommended. For some men, a periodic check of their testosterone level is also recommended after age 50, particularly if signs of low testosterone are apparent.

## Causes of Secondary Osteoporosis

### IMMOBILITY

Immobility may cause bone loss because of a lack of weight-bearing activities to stimulate bone formation and reduce or prevent bone loss. Immobility may occur from wearing a cast, being bedridden or general inactivity. Astronauts have been found to incur bone loss while living in space. This is due to their inability to bear weight in the absence of gravity. Without stress being applied directly to the bone, bone remodeling and normal bone formation will not occur.

### DISEASE

Several conditions may cause an imbalance in bone resorption and bone formation and subsequent bone loss. Even anorexia nervosa, bulimia or hormone imbalances (sometimes found in elite and extreme athletes) can lead to osteoporosis. Some of the more common diseases are described below. In all cases, measures to protect against bone loss should be implemented.

*Celiac disease* is a common medical condition that presents with abdominal complaints, such as diarrhea, and is associated with weight loss. It is a condition or disease of malabsorption (nutrients are not absorbed properly) caused by an abnormal immune reaction to gluten. Malabsorption of nutrients, such as calcium, results in bone loss and osteoporosis. Celiac disease can usually be diagnosed by a simple blood test, but some people may need a biopsy of the small bowel (by an upper endoscopy) to confirm this diagnosis.

*Malabsorption* of nutrients may also be caused by small bowel problems, prior stomach or bowel surgery, or by a lack of digestive enzymes.

*Crohn's disease* is an inflammatory bowel disease in which the mucosal lining of the intestines becomes swollen and develops deep sores (ulcers). The cause of Crohn's disease is unknown, but it is thought to be related to an immune system disorder. The digestive track may not absorb the nutrients as it should. Signs and symptoms of Crohn's disease include diarrhea and abdominal pain. Treatment is often high doses of prednisone or other glucocorticoids together with other drugs to reduce the inflammation and symptoms. Poor absorption of nutrients and the use of glucocorticoids contribute to bone loss.

*Cushing's disease* is a medical condition in which the body makes too much steroid hormones. This has a similar effect as giving too much prednisone and can result in dramatic bone loss and a high risk of serious fractures. Preventative therapy or medical treatment for osteoporosis should be considered.

*Hypogonadism* occurs when the body does not produce enough sex hormone, generally estrogen in women and testosterone in men. This is discussed in more detail in the next chapter.

*Hyperthyroidism* is a very common medical condition that presents with tremor, weight loss, anxiety symptoms and intolerance to heat. It leads to rapid turnover of bone and often results in osteoporosis. Taking too high a dose of thyroid supplements can do the same thing. Check with your doctor to make sure your thyroid level is normal. Have regular blood tests if you are taking thyroid medication.

*Anorexia nervosa* is a serious medical condition caused when teen girls or young women do not have adequate nutrition. A lack of calories and nutrients may result in low bone density. Without enough calcium, bones become thin and weak. Lack of nutrition causes both a lack of estrogen and less effective building of bone mass.

*Rheumatoid arthritis* is an inflammatory disorder that can affect the whole body, with its main symptoms seen in the joints. Many studies have shown that people with rheumatoid arthritis have lower bone density and an increased risk of fracture. Many factors influence bone remodeling, but it is difficult to identify which mechanism is responsible for the reduced bone mass. Gender, age, nutritional status, medications, disease severity and duration are among the factors that influence bone remodeling.

*Alcoholism* can lead to hormone deficiencies. This can result is reduced levels of testosterone in men and estrogen in women, increasing the risk of osteoporosis.

*Liver disease*, whether from alcohol abuse or some other cause, such as hepatitis, may also result in osteoporosis.

## DRUG-INDUCED BONE LOSS

Due to their effect on bone remodeling, certain drugs taken in low doses over long periods can lead to bone loss. Examples of commonly prescribed medications that interfere with bone formation over time are: glucocorticoids; thyroid hormones (in excessive doses); gonadotropin releasing hormones (used to treat endometriosis in women and prostate cancer in men); anti-androgen therapy (used to treat benign prostate enlargement, some acne, male pattern baldness and excessive hairiness); aromatase inhibitors (used to treat breast cancer and ovarian cancer); and some seizure or anticonvulsant drugs (phenytoin or Dilantin).

Glucocorticoid drugs are the most common and serious cause of drug-induced osteoporosis and subsequent fracture risk. Glucocorticoids are corticosteroids similar to those produced by the adrenal gland located just above the kidney. The most common glucocorticoid is prednisone, which is used to treat diseases associated with excessive inflammation.

Glucocorticoids play an important role in regulating water and salt in the body, blood sugar levels and metabolism and growth. They also slow the body's immune system and help to suppress allergic reactions. These medications are often used to treat arthritis, asthma and Crohn's disease. While they are important and may be potentially lifesaving with conditions such as asthma, they sometimes cause side effects, such as muscle wasting, weight gain and osteoporosis. The use of inhaled steroids may contribute to increased bone loss, although to a lesser extent the bone loss may be due to the severity of the underlying disease.

Many factors influence the cause of increased fracture risk for people on glucocorticoid therapy. At the cellular level, glucocorticoid therapy affects the function of osteoblasts (bone formation) and may contribute to the breakdown of bone micro-architecture (the bone structure). Glucocorticoid therapy has a negative effect on estrogen and testosterone. It also promotes muscle weakness.

As with other steroids, the length of time spent on glucocorticoids and the dosage taken are factors that will affect a person's risk of developing osteoporosis and resulting bone fractures. If you have been diagnosed with a chronic illness and if you are taking medication, such as prednisone, for a prolonged period (more than three months), consult your doctor about the impact of these medications on your risk of osteoporosis and fracture, and determine if an osteoporosis therapy is necessary.

There is good news, however. Research suggests that glucocorticoid-induced osteoporosis (GIO) can be prevented. Since bone loss is most rapid in the first six months of glucocorticoid use, preventive measures should begin immediately if therapy is expected to go beyond three months. The assessment of risk will include your baseline bone mineral density, how long you may be on therapy, your medical history (including any previous fractures), lifestyle, age and stage of life. All these may affect the course of prevention or treatment.

Proton pump inhibitors (PPI) are strong prescription antacid drugs. They are usually prescribed to treat conditions in which high levels of acid in the stomach lead to symptoms such as reflux or peptic ulcers. Earlier studies reported that proton pump inhibitors were associated with an increased risk of fractures and osteoporosis, but later research suggests this is not necessarily the case. Further research is needed.

Your doctor can help you to assess the ongoing benefits and risks of continued proton pump inhibitor therapy. As with most drugs, if you have been on a proton pump inhibitor for longer than a year, it is beneficial to review its value. In some situations, it may be possible to reduce or stop using the proton pump inhibitor to see if symptoms recur. Some doctors may switch you to an over-the-counter antacid, such as Tums (calcium carbonate), to assist with symptoms.

If it is determined that you should continue the proton pump inhibitor therapy, and you are taking calcium supplements, consider taking your calcium supplements with food. This will increase the acid levels in the stomach naturally. Higher stomach acid levels stimulated by the food will assist calcium absorption, especially with calcium carbonate. Another option may be to switch to calcium citrate, which is likely to be better absorbed when the stomach acid levels are lower, such as when taking a proton pump inhibitor.

Depo-Provera – the brand name for depot medroxyprogesterone acetate, a progestin hormone – is a medication that is often used in pre-menopausal women as a method of birth control. It is given by injection every few months. Depo-Provera decreases levels of estrogen and other hormones and, if used for prolonged periods, may cause bone loss or low bone density.

Although many people would prefer not to take medications, some medications may be necessary to help us enjoy the quality of life we desire. The medications we have discussed in this chapter are prescribed for a reason. The fact that they can also affect your bones suggests that you should consider ways to prevent bone loss associated with these medications. Do not lose sight of the benefit of a drug's treatment, such as preventing and treating a disease or condition, even though there are risks of side effects from the drug.

Make your choices based on your circumstances, your tolerance for the risk, your medical history and your lifestyle. Research has shown that there is widespread under-treatment of glucocorticoid-induced osteoporosis. So, if you are on glucocorticoid therapy or other medications that may increase the risk of fracture, it is also your responsibility to raise the issue with your doctor or healthcare provider and work with them to make sure your bones are being properly protected.

# CHAPTER 1 KEY POINTS

- Bone is a living tissue that is completely removed and replaced (known as remodeling) over a seven-year cycle.

- Most of us reach our peak bone mass by our late twenties or mid-thirties.

- Certain nutrients and hormones help maintain our bones.

- Lifestyle and genetics influence our bone health.

- The balance of bone building and bone removal (resorption) is affected by age.

- Some diseases and some medications adversely affect bone health. Steps should be taken to prevent or slow down bone loss if it is due to disease or medication.

# Menopause and Hormone Therapies

## MENOPAUSE

The word menopause comes from the Greek words "meno" meaning month and "pausis" meaning to halt. Menopause is often used more broadly to include peri-menopause, a less well defined period of time before menopause. Peri-menopause generally starts in the early forties when the menstrual cycle changes from its usual pattern to an irregular and somewhat unpredictable pattern that may last for several years. For North American women, the normal age range for menopause is 42 to 57 with the average age being 51.

In the previous chapter, we discussed post-menopausal bone loss of two to five percent caused by a decrease in estrogen. This chapter will discuss menopause, some issues and options for managing its symptoms, and the use of hormone therapies.

Menopause occurs because the ovaries no longer produce two specific hormones – estrogen and progesterone. Estrogen is the main sex hormone in women and essential to the menstrual cycle. One of the functions of progesterone is to balance the effects of estrogen. Hormone therapies refer to the use of estrogen and progesterone to treat menopause.

## Managing Symptoms

There are several things to consider when managing symptoms of menopause, such as making lifestyle changes, taking non-hormone and hormone prescription medications, and seeking complementary or alternative therapies. We know that a healthy lifestyle leads to a better outcome throughout peri-menopause. The natural loss of estrogen during menopause has an impact on lifestyle issues related to weight, diet, exercise, stress, alcohol and smoking. As women lose estrogen, the increased rate of bone loss becomes a concern. Adequate calcium and vitamin D supplementation along with regular, preferably weight-bearing exercises, are important in maintaining bone health.

Menopause management, which may include care provided by regulated practitioners of traditional Chinese medicine or regulated naturopaths, may vary depending on the healthcare provider's view of menopause. Some view menopause as a natural healthy occurrence that should not be interfered with. Others see it as a life situation that requires managing menopausal symptoms that can significantly affect a woman's health and quality of life. It is important to know your healthcare provider's views on menopause and therapies for menopausal symptoms. Keeping a diary of your symptoms will assist you in working with your doctor or healthcare provider to identify the best course of therapy for you. Make note of the date, time and the severity of your symptoms. Identify and rate the symptoms from one (minimal) to 10 (unbearable) at each occurrence.

Managing menopausal symptoms can be confusing and often controversial. Issues can arise over whether to use pharmaceutical drugs or compounded preparations or herbal remedies or to do nothing.

Hormone therapies manufactured by recognized pharmaceutical companies are regulated by federal or national licensing bodies. A hormone therapy may be prescribed to relieve some of the symptoms of menopause. Hormone therapy often provides some symptom relief as well as protection against bone loss and fracture. This protection stops when the hormone therapy stops. Based on your risk of osteoporosis, hormone therapy may be very appropriate during peri-menopause and menopause. Other treatments specific to reducing bone loss are discussed later in this book. You may wish to discuss these with your healthcare provider.

Compounded medications are manually prepared by a pharmacy based on the prescription requirements. The compounding industry and compounding preparations arose from special needs of patients, such as the need for a chewable alternative to a pill, a dye free option, or replacement of an older drug that is no longer made on a large scale. Some feel that although compounding is expensive, it is safer and more effective than commercial products, professing that the medications can be prepared exactly as the doctor ordered. Others say that compounded products have never been adequately tested and there is a not enough satisfactory evidence to support the belief that compounded products are better or safer. These people also have concerns that compounded products are unregulated for safety and purity, are costly and can be misleading to the consumer. In fact, the United States Food and Drug Administration (FDA) issued a warning in 2008 that compounded bio-identical hormone replacement therapy (BHRT) products "are unsupported by medical evidence, and are considered false and misleading by the agency" and any claims otherwise are misleading to women and healthcare providers.

Herbal remedies have been around for many years. As with the compounding industry, good long-term, double-blind, placebo-controlled studies for many herbal products have yet to be done.

You will find that most therapies come with their own benefits and side effects. All remedies that have an effect on the body can have an adverse effect or side effect. Do not be misled that a natural product has no side effects. Phytoestrogens are a plant source of estrogen-like molecules that have some effects like estrogen. Because the sources of phytoestrogen may vary, it is difficult to achieve a regular level of estrogen-like activity. Phytoestrogens have not yet been well studied to understand fully their risks and benefits, but they are likely to have estrogen-like effects and side effects.

Talk to friends or family members who have experienced menopause to identify what you might expect, recognizing that every woman's experience is unique. Be well informed and work with your healthcare provider to set your own goals and to develop the best management plan for you – individualized for your personal medical history, signs and symptoms.

Get to know the risks and benefits of any of your choices. Look for evidence-based information on efficacy, safety and bone health data. It may take a few months to sort out what is best for you. Your healthcare provider may have strong opinions on the choices you make, so be sure to discuss your choices with your provider before you start to experience any symptoms of menopause.

## HORMONE THERAPIES

Menopausal symptoms are generally treated one of three different ways:

- *Hormone therapy using a combination of estrogen and progesterone, or*

- *Estrogen therapy alone, or*

- *Progesterone therapy alone.*

The therapy you choose depends on your personal circumstances and your healthcare provider's view on menopause.

## Hormone Therapy

Hormone therapies were formerly referred to as hormone replacement therapy. The latter term is no longer used because the goal of the therapy is not to replace hormones that the body naturally produces, but to provide the lowest effective amount of hormones. Although hormone products are generally prescribed to help decrease menopausal symptoms, evidence shows that taking estrogen actually increases the amount of bone for the first few years of therapy. However, there are other effective therapies for osteoporosis that are more specific in improving bone with fewer risks and side effects. Bone protection is considered an additional benefit of hormone therapy.

Hormones can be used as an effective treatment for osteoporosis at any time, provided the benefits outweigh the risks. Once a hormone therapy is stopped, bone loss will return to its natural rate.

The 2002 Women's Health Initiative Study* points out a number of benefits and risks associated with therapies involving estrogen and progesterone or estrogen alone. The study showed that:

- *Hormone therapies were found to be effective in preventing bone loss and reduced the number of fractures by one-third. There were five fewer hip fractures in the 10,000 women followed for one year.*

- *Hormone therapies did not seem to cause more cases of breast cancer compared to the placebo (no drug) until after the fourth or fifth year of therapy. There were eight more breast cancer cases in 10,000 women followed for one year.*

- *Hormone therapies can significantly reduce colorectal cancer, which is the second most common cause of cancer death. However, the research on reducing colon cancer may not be sufficient to outweigh the risk of hormone therapies. There were six fewer colorectal cancers in 10,000 women followed for one year.*

- *Compared to the placebo, there were more cardiovascular events with hormone therapies. It is important to talk with your doctor about your own situation. There were seven more coronary heart disease events in 10,000 women followed for one year.*

- *Compared to the placebo, there were a higher number of blood clots and strokes in the group receiving hormone therapies. There were 18 more clot events and seven more stroke events in 10,000 women followed for one year.*

- *Hormone therapies taken even up to seven years do not shorten lifespan.*

- *Further research needs to be done to determine if there is a benefit using hormone therapies for dementia.*

*\* The Women's Health Initiative was a 15-year study of 161,808 women aged 50-79. Sponsored by the National Institutes of Health and the National Heart, Lung and Blood Institute, the study focused on strategies for preventing heart disease, breast and colorectal cancer and osteoporosis in post-menopausal women. These chronic diseases are the major causes of death, disability and frailty in older women. Learn more about this study online.*

A hormone therapy prescribed for one or more of these reasons is usually taken for less than five years of continuous use.

If a woman chooses a hormone therapy, the best time to start may be during the peri-menopausal and early post-menopause period to help reduce common symptoms of menopause. Hot flashes (also known as flushes), night sweats, frequent urination, insomnia, irritability, vaginal dryness, breast tenderness, depression, changes in sexual desire and bone loss are some of the symptoms of menopause.

Hormone therapy for menopausal symptom control is not usually recommended until the symptoms disappear or after five years. Women over 60 are not usually started on a hormone therapy. With the availability of other drug therapies proven to reduce fractures, hormone therapies, which may cause long term side effects, are not first choice or first-line therapy in the United States or Canada for the prevention or treatment of osteoporosis.

Hormone therapies can be taken in several forms: pill, monthly injection, skin patch or gel, vaginal cream, ring or tablet. Some estrogen therapies that have been approved for preventing osteoporosis in post-menopausal women are Climara, Estrace, Estraderm, Estratab, Ogen, Ortho-Est, Premarin and Vivelle. Their effect on bone will vary depending on dosage, how the drug is prepared and how it is administered.

However, not all forms of estrogen therapies have received approval by the Food and Drug Administration in the United States or by the Therapeutic Products Directorate in Canada. Sometimes these medications are compounded products.

Hormone treatments can be taken in a number of ways. Depending on your personal situation, estrogen, which is used to correct a deficiency of estrogen, may be taken each day of the month (this is the usual recommendation), or it may be taken the first day after menstrual bleeding for up to 21 days out of 28, or it could be taken for 24 or 25 days in a month.

Progesterone used daily at a low dose is the usual recommendation for continuous combined therapy. However, alternatives may be to take progesterone for 10 or 14 days a month for cyclical therapy or take it only every second or third month for 10 or 14 days.

Doctors may also recommend that estrogen and a small dose of progesterone be taken together every day. This method is easy to remember and usually means that there is no vaginal bleeding. Research on the effect of continuous, long-term estrogen as well as an estrogen and progesterone combination is still ongoing. Speak with your doctor or pharmacist to help determine the best regimen for you.

A common mistake is choosing the wrong dose of hormone. Women are generally advised to take the lowest effective dose, starting at 0.3mg conjugated estrogen daily or, in the case of the estradiol, 0.5mg daily. Hormone treatments are proven to increase bone mineral density. Some experts feel that higher dosages of hormone therapies are more effective with severe osteoporosis. However, the side effects of estrogen are such that a higher dose might not be recommended.

Women who smoke do not benefit from oral estrogen. Ideally, you should not smoke. Estrogen absorbed from a skin patch is not affected by smoking.

Side effects of hormone therapies can include:

- *Monthly vaginal bleeding from the monthly withdrawal of hormone*
- *Salt and water retention (bloating)*
- *Breast swelling and tenderness*
- *Increased risk of breast cancer*
- *Increased risk of thrombosis (blood clot or stroke)*
- *Increased risk of heart disease if started later (after age 65)*

Although the side effects of estrogen may seem alarming, remember to establish your personal risk based on your medical history compared to your risk of developing osteoporosis.

Women who have any of the following health issues should discuss the risks and benefits of hormone therapy with their doctor and be given individualized treatment for their medical situation, which may include:

- *High blood pressure*
- *Estrogen-related migraine headaches*
- *Gall bladder or pancreas problems*
- *Obesity*
- *High blood sugar (diabetes)*

Hormone therapies for someone with high blood sugar or diabetes is not a contraindication. Some research shows a reduction of type 2 diabetes in women on estrogen and progesterone therapy. This is potentially an added benefit of the hormone therapy, but would not be the primary reason someone would be treated with a hormone therapy.

A monthly breast self-examination and an annual breast examination by your doctor are important for every woman over the age of 50 and especially for those on a hormone therapy. Some experts encourage women 40 to 79 to have mammograms every 24 months. Ask your doctor about when and how often you should have a mammogram.

Discuss with your healthcare provider the positive and negative effects of taking estrogen, the recommended dose, the duration of use, how possible side effects should be monitored and how these relate to your own medical history.

## Estrogen Therapy Alone

If you have had a hysterectomy (removal of the uterus), you are no longer at risk of endometriosis or endometrial cancer, so estrogen therapy alone can be used to control menopausal symptoms. Continuous estrogen without progesterone may be given orally or by using gels, vaginal creams or a skin patch.

As a source of continuous estrogen, a vaginal cream or ring is helpful in controlling menopausal vaginal symptoms, but they have not been proven to have any major benefit on bone health.

## Progesterone Therapy

Most experts do not believe that progesterone, if used alone, prevents osteoporosis.

Unless they have had a hysterectomy, women on estrogen therapy should consider progesterone therapy in combination to decrease the risk of endometrial cancer. Benefits may include:

- *Improved quality of sleep, only if the natural progesterone Prometrium, which is made from plant sources, is used*

- *Reduced risk of cancer of the uterus associated with estrogen therapy*

- *Decreased risk of endometrial cancer associated with the estrogen in hormone therapies to below the natural risk*

Progesterone can be given orally, transdermally (skin patch), using an intrauterine device (IUD) or by injection. Common oral progesterones include medroxyprogesterone, norethindrone and micronized progesterone. Progesterone therapy is usually administered in one of two ways: cyclic ( given 10 to 14 days each month) or continuous (given each day of the week).

Continuous or cyclic use of progesterone stops monthly menstruation, but it may occasionally cause "breakthrough bleeding" (spotting). Continuous use of progesterone will help to reduce the risk of endometrial cancer. There is some evidence that progesterone decreases the good or positive effects of estrogens on the lipid profile, which is used to assess your risk for various heart conditions. Be sure to discuss this with your healthcare provider in consideration of your family history and cardiovascular risk.

Progesterone, like estrogen, may also contribute to breast cancer. This needs further study. It may also cause breast tenderness and increase the risk of blood clots.

Menopause is not the only reason why the menstrual cycle may stop. Extreme athletics, pregnancy, radiation or surgical removal of the ovaries can also lead to a change in your menstrual cycle. If your menstrual cycle stops, do not assume that you are in beginning stages of menopause. As with any changes in your menstrual cycle, it is important to consult with your doctor or other healthcare provider to identify or confirm why these changes are happening in your body.

Be your own best advocate. Learn all you can from trustworthy sources and then talk with your doctor or healthcare provider about your personal medical history and bone health status.

# CHAPTER 2 KEY POINTS

- Estrogen plays a significant role in preventing bone loss.

- Women can take steps to slow bone loss through adequate calcium, vitamin D and exercise.

- Your healthcare provider may have strong opinions on how to treat symptoms of menopause. Be sure to discuss your options with your provider before you start to experience any symptoms.

- Identify and rate the severity of symptoms from one to 10 at each occurrence in order to help manage the symptoms.

- Hormone therapies may provide relief for some menopausal symptoms.

- Hormone treatments for menopausal symptom control is usually recommended until the symptoms disappear or around five years.

- Post-menopausal women may experience rapid bone loss during the first six years after menopause.

- Estrogen treatment can be used as an effective treatment for osteoporosis at any time, provided the benefits outweigh the risks

- Once estrogen treatment is stopped, the rate of bone loss will return to its natural rate.

- The use of hormone therapy for more than five years can lead to higher risks compared to benefits.

- If you are post-menopausal and at moderate or high risk of osteoporosis or fracture, there are more effective medication options than estrogen for reducing fracture risk.

# CHAPTER 3

# Testosterone, Andropause and Bone Loss

## CALLING ALL MEN

Historically, osteoporosis research focused primarily on women. Consequently, less was known about prevention and treatment of osteoporosis in men. At one time, it was believed that the decline in men's bone health lagged 10 years behind women. Research now tells us that the lag time is only four to five years behind women.

Today, we know that osteoporosis does not only affect women; aging males should also be assessed for osteoporosis and fracture risk. The amount of men's testosterone declines with age. It is estimated that 10 percent of men over the age of 50 experience symptoms of low testosterone. Low testosterone is one of several risk factors for osteoporosis and fracture in men. This chapter will review hypogonadism and andropause (or androgen deficiency in the aging male as some refer to it) in relation to the prevention and treatment of bone loss in men.

Research suggests that osteoporosis in men is a common disease. It is estimated that one in eight men over the age of 50 suffer from low bone density or osteoporosis. By age 50, a man has a 13 percent chance of a fracture as a result of weak bones. By age 60, that risk increases to 25 percent. Thirty-five percent of all hip fractures occur among elderly males.

Androgens are the male hormones secreted by the gonads (testicles) and, to a small degree, the adrenal glands. Testosterone, the main androgen, is a male hormone responsible for secondary sexual features, such as musculature and strength, low voice, a beard and sex drive or libido. It affects many of the body's systems including the brain, heart and skeleton.

Hypogonadism is a condition in which the body does not produce enough sex hormones. Hypogonadism is derived from "hypo" meaning low, "gonad" meaning sex organ and "ism" meaning condition. In men, hypogonadism may be an age-related condition or due to damage to the pituitary (a gland in the brain that controls and releases hormones in the body). Hypogonadism may be the result of certain prostate cancer therapies, the removal of testicles, or the result of the testicles being normal but functioning improperly.

## TESTOSTERONE LEVELS

The decline in the male hormone testosterone with age is gradual, unlike the rapid decline in estrogen experienced by females during peri-menopause or at menopause. Moreover, a significant decline in testosterone levels is neither universal nor experienced by all aging males.

Andropause, sometimes referred to as male menopause, is also termed androgen deficiency in the aging male (ADAM) or hypogonadism. Generally, andropause is the result of low testosterone and can reach a point where the level of testosterone is so low that it causes medical symptoms that require correcting. The word andropause comes from the Greek words "andros" meaning men and "pausis" meaning to halt. This is not quite an accurate term because the testosterone production does not actually halt or stop, it simply declines gradually to a point that may cause some unwelcome signs and symptoms.

Signs and symptoms of low testosterone can be vague and can vary significantly from one man to another. Some will describe the feeling, saying: "I used to be a jock and now I am a couch potato." Symptoms can be broadly grouped as:

- *Low sex drive*

- *Decreased frequency of erections*

- *Emotional, psychological and behavior changes*

- *Muscle aches and reduced muscle strength*
- *Increased upper and central body fat*
- *Decline in general well-being and energy level*
- *Mental fatigue and reduced ability to concentrate*

The following questions* can help you to determine if you may be suffering from low testosterone. If you answer yes to questions 1 and 7 or yes to any three questions, discuss these symptoms with your doctor or healthcare provider.

1. *Do you have decreased interest in sex (libido)?*
2. *Do you have a lack of energy?*
3. *Do you have a decrease in strength and/or endurance?*
4. *Have you lost height?*
5. *Have you noticed a decreased enjoyment in life?*
6. *Are you sad and/or grumpy?*
7. *Are your erections less strong?*
8. *Have you noticed a recent deterioration in your ability to play a sport you used to play well?*
9. *Are you falling asleep after dinner?*
10. *Has there been a recent deterioration in your work performance?*

Your healthcare provider may suspect these symptoms are caused by something other than low testosterone, such as depression. Your healthcare provider may say: "You are getting older, what do you expect?" or "At your age, you will have more aches and pains" or "You can't expect to do what you did at age 30."

Since we all experience days when we "feel old," these statements may be true on some days. However, if these feelings persist over time, keep a record. Review the questionnaire and your symptoms (including a description of the symptoms and

* *These questions were developed by John E. Morley, MB, BCh at St. Louis University Medical Center, St. Louis, Missouri. They are reproduced here with permission from Dr. John E. Morley (2010).*

the time of day they occur) with your healthcare provider. Blood tests that measure the level of testosterone may be necessary to help assess your situation. Your healthcare provider may order blood tests, such as a free testosterone level, sex hormone binding globulin (SHBG) level, and/or total testosterone level (see the glossary for an explanation).

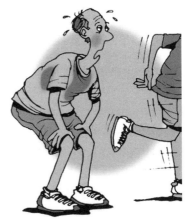

**A decrease in endurance may be sign of low testosterone.**

An osteoporosis and fracture risk assessment together with review and discussion of the questionnaire with your healthcare provider are important to assess your bone health. Calculate your 10-year fracture risk using FRAX (see Chapter 9). If you have had a fracture or have a low bone mineral density measurement, your healthcare provider may require laboratory tests to identify the cause of the bone loss. The test results will help to more accurately identify the cause of the bone loss and the appropriate treatment. The increased risk of fracture may be from primary hypogonadism where the problem originates from declining levels of testosterone or it might be from secondary hypogonadism where the testicles are normal but function improperly. In either case, the bone loss must be managed.

Men who receive anti-androgen therapy, such as cyproterone acetate, are at increased risk of bone loss and possibly fracture. Other secondary risk factors are discussed in Chapter 1.

The approach to prevention of bone loss includes having a daily intake of 1,000mg to 1,200mg elemental calcium (total amount combined from diet and supplements) and up to 2,000IU vitamin D in men over 50 years of age, and doing weight-bearing exercises. When symptoms warrant and a doctor has identified a significantly low testosterone level, testosterone replacement therapy for the male with hypogonadism may be used.

# TESTOSTERONE REPLACEMENT THERAPY

As previously mentioned, androgens are the male hormones secreted by the gonads (testicles) and, to a small degree, the adrenal glands. Androgens have important effects on the bones. Testosterone, the main androgen, is thought to reduce the rate of bone breakdown by acting as an anti-resorptive.

Small studies have shown improvement in bone density among men with hypogonadism taking testosterone replacement therapy for three years. It has also been reported that unless the testosterone level is low in a man at risk of fracture, supplementing with additional testosterone will not necessarily increase bone density or prevent fracture. However, those with significantly low testosterone may benefit from testosterone replacement therapy.

Testosterone replacement therapy should not be confused with treatments used for erectile dysfunction – for example taking sildenafil (Viagra), tadalafil (Cialis) or vardenafil (Levitra). The treatments for erectile dysfunction help to produce erections in men with erectile dysfunction, regardless of testosterone level and do not prevent bone loss or fractures. Men with low testosterone levels or who experience hypogonadism may find testosterone replacement can help slow down bone loss and improve well-being, libido, sex drive and erections. Testosterone replacement therapy and treatments used for erectile dysfunction are very different and should not be confused with each other or used interchangeably.

## Benefits of Testosterone Replacement Therapy

For men with low testosterone levels, testosterone replacement therapy may help to improve associated symptoms and positively impact overall health and well-being. Testosterone replacement therapy can also prevent or reduce long term risks of hypogonadism. Research is showing that low levels of androgens, such as testosterone, have important effects on our bones, especially in relation to bone loss. We have discussed that as a man ages, his testosterone levels decline. Low levels of testosterone put men at a higher risk of developing osteoporosis and having a less than optimal quality of life. Questions to ask are: What is the risk for future fracture? Should the low testosterone be treated?

Testosterone replacement therapies are commonly available as injectable testosterone cypionate (Depo-testosterone) or testosterone enanthate (Delatestrayl), as a patch or gel (Androderm, Androgel) or as oral testosterone undecanoate (Andriol). Oral forms of testosterone may be associated with a higher risk of liver toxicity.

Your healthcare provider should closely monitor your response to treatment, ensuring that the dose used is suitable and that regular blood tests for side effects are done.

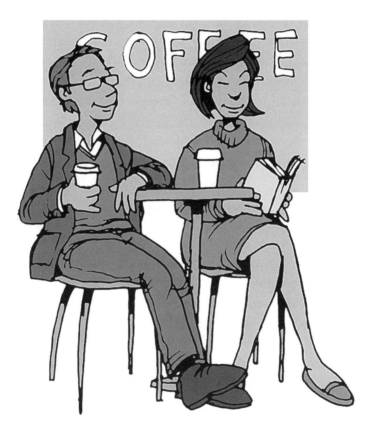

## Possible Side Effects of Testosterone Replacement Therapy

- *Liver disorders*
- *Increase in red blood cells*
- *Prostate enlargement*
- *Suppression of good cholesterol*
- *Acne*
- *Fluctuation in mood*
- *Fluid retention*

The risk of testosterone replacement therapy should be considered on an individual basis. Discuss with your doctor.

Contraindications (reasons for not taking a therapy) for testosterone replacement therapy include current or past breast or prostate cancer, sleep apnea (a temporary cessation in breathing during sleep) and liver conditions. While there are concerns about the risk of prostate cancer, testosterone supplementation research has not provided a definitive answer.

The risks of testosterone replacement therapy should be considered on an individual basis. Discuss the treatment with your doctor to establish your personal risk based on your medical history, risk of hypoganadal symptoms, future fracture risk, wellness and quality of life issues.

## OTHER TREATMENTS FOR OSTEOPOROSIS IN MEN

Bisphosphonates have been studied in men with low bone density and have shown to increase bone density compared to placebo. Three bisphosphonates currently approved by the regulatory authorities in the United States and Canada for the prevention or treatment of osteoporosis in men are: alendronate, risedronate, and zoledronic acid (see Chapter 11). The parathyroid hormone terriparatide is approved by the same regulatory authorities to increase bone mass in men at high risk of fracture.

It is important to know that studies have shown that osteoporosis treatments for women reduce fractures. To date, there have been no similar studies for men. More studies are urgently needed for men with osteoporosis. In the meantime, men and their doctors should assume that treatments will improve bone density and provide results similar to women.

## MONITOR YOUR THERAPY

Current recommendations for screening, monitoring and treating men with low testosterone include prostate-specific antigen (PSA), other blood tests and a digital rectal examination before and during testosterone therapy. Ask for a copy of your test results for your own medical files.

Talk with your doctor about the usefulness of a PSA test. Some experts strongly recommend regular PSA tests and are concerned about rising values as related to early detection of possible prostate cancer. Others argue that assessing PSA levels will not affect the management of prostate health and the tests may lead to further unnecessary or inappropriate tests.

Low testosterone in the aging male is a problem. As well as contributing to bone loss, low testosterone can lead to a decrease in health and well-being. Experts continue to debate the risks and benefits of treatment. Men should talk with their healthcare providers about their opinions and views on aging and quality of life. Remember, low testosterone is not the only cause of bone loss in men. Depending on the identified cause of bone loss, you and your doctor or healthcare provider should discuss other treatment options for osteoporosis.

Much research is still required to identify which risk factors are the most significant in men and which treatments are best for men at risk of developing osteoporosis.

## CHAPTER 3 KEY POINTS

- Osteoporosis in men is common.

- Men can take steps to slow bone loss through adequate calcium, vitamin D and exercise.

- Testosterone declines as men get older. Some may have significant signs and symptoms of low testosterone such as persistent lack of energy, decreased interest in sex, less strong erections, sadness or grumpiness.

- Hypogonadism (low testosterone) is one of several important risk factors for bone loss in men.

- Thirty-five percent of hip fractures occur among elderly males.

- Testosterone replacement therapy may be recommended for men with hypogonadism to prevent bone loss.

- Bisphosphonates and parathyroid hormones are effective therapies for osteoporosis in men.

# PART TWO

# Osteoporosis Prevention

Calcium

Vitamin D and Other Vitamins and Minerals

The Importance of Exercising and Safe Movement

Exercises

## CHAPTER 4

# Calcium

In Part Two of *The Osteoporosis Book* we will discuss non-pharmacological ways to slow down – although not prevent – the onset of osteoporosis through diet and exercise. We identify foods that are high in calcium or that affect the absorption of calcium; we offer suggestions on how to adjust your diet to improve calcium absorption; and we discuss the value of vitamin D and other vitamins and minerals. If you are unable to get enough dietary calcium and vitamin D from food, you will learn about supplements that you might be able to use. Finally, we provide exercises and tips to maintain bone health.

## DIET AND BONE HEALTH

A well-balanced diet should provide your body with the necessary fats, carbohydrates, proteins, water, mineral salts and vitamins. National daily food guides are designed to help ensure that all nutrients are obtained in a proper balance to meet our basic nutritional needs. Nutrients do not work on their own, but with other nutrients. Carbohydrates, fats and proteins provide the body with the energy and building blocks it needs. Electrolytes, water, vitamins and minerals are important for the cellular build-up and break-down that occurs in the body. Not all foods are equal in the nutrition they offer, so some foods receive more attention in food guides. Food guides, such as the United States Department of Agriculture's MyPyramid Food Guidance System and Health Canada's Canada Food Guide are available online, through your library, from healthcare providers, and especially from a registered dietitian or health clinics.

Your body has several built-in regulating mechanisms. A change in one thing will likely affect something else. The change may be for the better or worse, but the result of the change may take months or years to show up. Consider how slowly the body builds bone. In some parts of our body, bone keeps building into our thirties. If we maintained an optimal well-balanced healthy diet during those years and got plenty of exercise, the risk of developing osteoporosis would be reduced.

Minerals (such as calcium, phosphorus and magnesium) and vitamins (such as vitamin D, vitamin A and vitamin K) are important in bone health. With the possible exception of vitamin D, other minerals and vitamins are more than adequately covered in a varied, well-balanced, healthy diet, provided you are absorbing the nutrients.

## CALCIUM

The body needs calcium for:

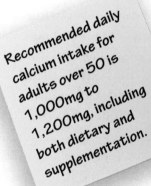

- *Strong teeth and bones*

- *Nerve and muscle function*

- *Maintaining cell permeability (the passage of fluids through the cell walls)*

- *Regulating blood pressure and maintaining normal heart rate and rhythm*

- *Blood clotting*

If our daily diet does not include enough calcium, or if calcium is not absorbed properly in our bodies, our blood calcium levels decrease. The parathyroid gland, which is responsible for maintaining blood calcium levels, will then send out more parathyroid hormone to release more calcium from bones in order to improve calcium levels. If blood calcium levels remain low over several years, parathyroid hormone may cause calcium to be taken constantly from the bone. Over a long period of time, bones can become brittle and are at greater risk of fracturing.

Calcium has an important role in the prevention and treatment of osteoporosis. The daily recommended amount of calcium in an average person's diet is between 1,000mg and 1,200mg, depending on age, gender and medical history. About 75 percent of the calcium in an average diet is from dairy products. Eating a regular amount of calcium-rich foods is the best way to ensure that calcium is always available when your body needs it. Many people find it difficult to maintain a diet that meets the recommended calcium intake.

Dairy products are the richest sources of calcium. Fortified rice or soy beverages contain the equivalent amount of calcium as found in milk – 8oz/250ml equals about 320mg of calcium. For people who have trouble tolerating milk, adding the enzyme lactase to milk helps break down the milk sugar and may improve the ability to digest milk. If you have an allergy to milk products or choose to avoid dairy products, discuss your diet and need for calcium supplements with your healthcare provider. Calcium supplements and non-dairy foods containing calcium are discussed later in this chapter.

The body's calcium requirements vary with age, lifestyle and general health. Certain foods, diseases and medications can affect the amount of calcium the stomach and intestines are able to draw into the bloodstream from the food you eat. Certain components of food, particularly oxalates and phytates, may result in a decrease in calcium absorption.

Any of the following can result in the depletion of some nutrients in your body. If any of these apply to you, consider adjusting your diet or taking supplements:

- *Not eating a well-balanced diet. Older people may eat too little and have a poor diet (such as just taking tea and toast) and younger people may be constantly dieting or be anorexic.*

- *A lifestyle that includes high stress and smoking.*

- *Food allergies that prevent you from getting the necessary nutrients.*

- *The body does not process nutrients normally.*

- *Glands that over-produce or under-produce hormones that impact calcium levels.*

- *Digestive problems, such as celiac or Crohn's disease, that cause malabsorption.*

- *Medications that impact the digestive system, which can cause malabsorption of nutrients.*

*Certain components of food, particularly oxalates and phytates, may result in a decrease in calcium absorption.*

When too little calcium is available, the body will rob the bones of the calcium it needs in order to maintain calcium levels in the blood. Over time, bones may become thinner. While most people recognize the importance of dairy products as a source of calcium, many are not aware of other sources of calcium. Calcium supplements, for example, may be required if you cannot maintain the minimum recommended calcium levels through your diet.

If you are at increased risk for developing osteoporosis, discuss with your doctor or healthcare provider the possibility of increasing your calcium intake. If you have a history of kidney stones, precautions should be considered. A good work-up or medical assessment from your doctor or specialist should help to rule out any underlying causes or factors that impact how much calcium you should take.

## CALCIUM INTAKE

Use the checklist below to give you an approximate calculation of your dietary calcium intake. If you are low or borderline, you may want to do a more detailed calculation with your doctor, nurse practitioner or registered dietitian. Websites of national osteoporosis organizations and most dairy foundations also offer methods to calculate calcium. Libraries and your healthcare providers also have charts to calculate your calcium intake.

## Quick Calcium Intake Check List

A simple way to calculate your calcium intake is to:

- *List all the foods you eat in a day. For a more accurate reflection, list the foods you eat over three days and include a weekend when your diet may be different from your usual weekdays.*

- *List the foods in easily measurable amounts, such as cups, ounces or milliliters.*

- *Use the food charts on the following pages (or any other food chart) and list the milligrams (mg) of calcium in each food. Some foods do not contain significant amounts of calcium and are not listed here. Consider the amount of calcium that these foods contribute as a bonus to your daily calcium intake.*

- *Add up the amounts. Be sure to check serving sizes and milligrams, then adjust as necessary. Compare your amounts with the recommendations for your age group.*

When counting your calcium intake, consider both dietary intake and supplements. Do not forget to include multivitamins.

Although research on the recommended amount of calcium required per day is ongoing, the National Osteoporosis Foundation and Osteoporosis Canada recommends:

| Age | Calcium mg/day |
| --- | --- |
| 4-8 | 800mg |
| 9-18 | 1,300mg |
| 19-50 | 1,000mg |
| 50+ | 1,200mg* |

Experts suggest the best way to get calcium is through a balanced diet and, if necessary, supplements. Many suggest the safe upper limit for a total calcium intake should not exceed 1,500mg to 1,800mg per day unless you have malabsorption issues or unless

* *Many adults only consume 300mg to 700mg per day. A well balanced non-dairy diet often contains 300mg of calcium. Some experts recommend up to 1,500mg daily.*

your doctor or dietitian recommends otherwise. Research is also showing that individuals over the age of 50 who have sufficient vitamin D intake require a total daily calcium intake of between 800mg and 1,200mg per day. If your primary source of calcium is from foods other than dairy products, you may need to consume a large quantity of these foods in order to meet the recommended daily requirement of calcium.

**If your intake of calcium and vitamin D is inadequate, intake of caffeine, soft drinks and foods high in protein and fiber become much more relevant. These drinks and foods decrease the amount of calcium in your body.**

More calcium is not always better. The calcium you get from the food you eat is best. However, if food does not provide you with an adequate amount of calcium, you may need a calcium supplement.

While calcium is important, too much calcium may be harmful. Some studies* have shown a link between high calcium intake (diet plus supplements) and an increased risk of heart complications and other studies showed no such link. The Women's Health Initiative (referred to in Chapter 2) did not confirm a link between calcium supplements and increased heart complications, but it did show a slight increase in the risk of kidney stones. Further research is ongoing to identify the optimal daily calcium intake.

The following charts cluster foods into categories based on their calcium content. It is important to know the general amount of calcium rather than the specific amount; hence the figures are in round numbers rather than specific amounts. An 8oz/250ml glass of milk contains about 320mg of calcium and 100IU of

*The Calcium Supplementation Study in New Zealand (authored by M.J. Bolland and colleagues) compared a relatively small group of 700 women taking calcium supplements to 700 women taking a placebo (sugar pills) over a five-year period. The researchers found that the women taking calcium supplements had a higher incidence of heart attack. The study was carried out to see if calcium supplementation would provide benefit to the cardiovascular (heart and blood vessel) system.*

vitamin D. Similarly, an 8oz/250ml glass of fortified rice and soy milk also contains about 320mg of calcium. Therefore, drinking two glasses of milk a day is a good start toward meeting your daily calcium requirements. If vegetables are your main source of calcium, you will need to eat a lot more vegetables than what is recommended in these charts in order to get the recommended daily requirement of calcium.

## 300 - 500MG OF CALCIUM PER SERVING

| Food | Estimated Serving |
|---|---|
| Beans: Black | 1 cup/250ml |
| Bok Choy: Cooked | 1 cup/250ml |
| Cheese: Brick, Caraway, Colby, Edam | 1.5oz/45g |
| Cheese: Ricotta (skimmed milk) | 1 cup/250ml |
| Cheese: Farmers, Swiss | 1.5oz/45g |
| Macaroni and Cheese | 1 cup/250ml |
| Milk: Fortified Rice or Soy | 1 cup/250ml |
| Milk: Evaporated, Undiluted (2%, skim, whole) | 1 cup/250ml |
| Milk: Powdered Skim | 4tbsp/60ml |
| Milk: Buttermilk, Chocolate | 1 cup/250ml |
| Milk Shake | 1 cup/250ml |
| Sardines with Bones | 3oz/90g |
| Tofu: in Calcium Sulfate | 1 cup/250ml |
| Yogurt: Plain, Skim | 6oz/180ml |

## 200 - 300MG OF CALCIUM PER SERVING

| Food | Estimated Serving |
|---|---|
| Cheese: Blue, Feta, Mozzarella | 1.5oz/45g |
| Cheese: Parmesan | 3tbsp/100g |
| Cheese: Processed | 1.5oz/45g |
| Ice Cream Sundae | 1 cup/250ml |
| Milk: Powdered, Whole | 4tbsp/60ml |
| Salmon: Canned, Drained, with bones | 0.5 cup/125ml |

## 100 - 200MG OF CALCIUM PER SERVING

| Food | Estimated Serving |
|------|-------------------|
| Almonds | 1.5oz/45g |
| Baked Beans with Tomato Sauce | 1 cup/250ml |
| Brazil Nuts | 0.5 cup/125ml |
| Broccoli Cooked | 1 cup/250ml |
| Cheese: Cottage 4%, skim | 1 cup/250ml |
| Chile Con Carne and Beans | 1 cup/250ml |
| Cream of Wheat Cooked | 1 cup/250ml |
| Custard Baked | 0.5 cup/125ml |
| Custard Pie | 1 wedge |
| English Muffin with Egg, Cheese and Bacon | 1 |
| Figs: Dried, 5 medium | 3oz/90g |
| Ice Cream | 0.75 cup/185ml |
| Kale | 0.5 cup/125ml |
| Lobster | 3oz/90g |
| Molasses: Blackstrap/Cooking | 1tbsp/15ml |
| Pizza with Cheese | 1 piece |
| Pudding: Instant, Rice, Tapioca | 0.5 cup/125ml |
| Sesame Seeds | 0.5 cup/125ml |
| Shrimp | 28 med. size |
| Soup: Cream of Chicken, Mushroom, Tomato | 1 cup/250ml |
| Soy Beans | 1 cup/250ml |
| Spaghetti and Meat Sauce | 1 cup/250ml |
| White Beans | 1 cup/250ml |

## Foods that Rob Bones of Calcium

Some foods can rob your bones of calcium. Calcium robbers are foods that are high in oxalates and phytates. Regular servings of these foods are good for you and do not pose a threat. However, when taken in large quantities, these foods may interfere or block absorption of calcium. Do not stop eating these foods, but try to avoid eating them with foods you depend on for calcium. Alternatively, you can increase your calcium intake at the time you eat these foods.

Use these tips to help manage these issues:

- *Foods containing oxalates, such as rhubarb, spinach, beet greens and Swiss chard, carry valuable minerals and vitamins that your body needs.*
  *Tip: Eat a variety of vegetables, especially dark green, leafy vegetables, such as collard, kale, mustard and turnip greens, to balance out the oxalates.*

- *Foods containing phytates, such as pita bread, navy beans, kidney beans, peas, and wheat and bran cereals, have valuable nutrients.*
  *Tip: Increase your calcium intake in other ways when you eat these foods, by adding, for example, a slice of cheese or a glass of milk.*

- *Too much protein may increase your calcium loss through your kidneys, but the body needs protein to function effectively.*
  *Tip: Eat small amounts of protein with every meal rather than one large serving a day.*

- *Fiber can move food quickly through the digestive track, but you need fiber for heart health and regularity, so fibre should be a part of a well-balanced diet.*
  *Tip: Do not rely only on the amount of calcium eaten with a high-fibre meal to provide the calcium you need. Remember, the fiber from your cereal is good for you, but only a small amount of the calcium from milk will be absorbed when milk is eaten with a high-fiber breakfast cereal. Drink another glass of milk a few hours later to ensure you get the calcium you need.*

- *In addition to contributing to high blood pressure, the salt or sodium found in the table salt that you add to your meals and the processed foods you eat may cause calcium loss through your kidneys. Be sure to read the labels. More than 90 percent of the average person's sodium comes from additives found in processed and fast foods. The food industry is working with governments to remove the salt added unnecessarily to foods. There is evidence to suggest calcium loss through urine may be increased with excess salt intake.*
  *Tip: Be aware of your salt intake. Try a different spice to modify flavor.*

- *Caffeine increases the loss of calcium through the urine.*
  *Tip: Replace coffee, cola drinks and some energy drinks with non-caffeine beverages, such as flavored milk or hot chocolate. The amount of caffeine in chocolate is not enough to affect the amount of calcium lost in urine. Tea has an insignificant impact on calcium intake. If you must drink coffee or other caffeine beverages, avoid drinking more than three cups per day. To increase the calcium intake, add milk.*

Remember, if you are eating large amounts of food that reduce calcium absorption or increase the loss of calcium, try to balance or replace the lost calcium.

## Increase Dietary Calcium

A well-balanced diet is essential for a healthy body. It is important to consider the foods that can block your calcium absorption or rob you of calcium during digestion, so be sure to increase your calcium intake while also consuming these foods. Here are some easy ways to increase your intake of calcium.

### ADD:

- *Dry-milk powder to fluid milk, one-third cup of powder per one cup milk will double the calcium content (one teaspoon contains about 50mg of calcium)*

- *Grated cheese to casseroles, vegetable dishes, popcorn, toast*

- *A slice of cheese to sandwiches*

- A cup of cooked soybeans to soup
- Cooked soybeans to mayonnaise and seasoning to make a sandwich spread

**SUBSTITUTE:**
- Low-fat milk for water in most soups, drink mixes and baked products
- Yogurt for sour cream
- Yogurt and dry milk powder for mayonnaise
- Desserts, such as rice puddings, tapioca, custards and bread puddings, for pastries, cakes and other foods high in fat.
- Skim ricotta cheese for cottage cheese
- Soybeans for other kinds of beans in a recipe

**GENERAL:**
- Use tofu that has been prepared with calcium sulfate rather than calcium salt or magnesium (read the label).
- Drink milk shakes or hot milk flavored with cinnamon, cloves, almond extract or a small amount of decaffeinated coffee instead of soft drinks or regular coffee.
- Use roasted soybeans to enhance a snack recipe.
- Drink orange juice fortified with calcium and vitamin D.

## Understanding Food Labels

When reading a label, look for the calcium content. The percentage (%) of Daily Value (DV) or percentage (%) of Recommended Daily Intake (RDI) noted on a label is generally based on approximately 1,000mg of calcium per day. So, a label stating "calcium 10 percent" would mean that one serving contains 100mg of calcium is in one serving of that item. Be sure to read the label and note the amount of a "serving size."

# High Calcium Diets

People who have diets high in calcium, particularly diets that are high in dairy products, may encounter problems. Problems include lactose intolerance, constipation and high fat intake.

## LACTOSE INTOLERANCE

To be properly digested, milk sugar (lactose) in dairy products must be broken down by the body. The body produces the enzyme lactase to break down the milk sugar. Some people are not able to produce enough of this enzyme. When milk sugar is not broken down and digested, the result may be bloating, abdominal cramping, diarrhea and gas.

### Tips:

- *Eat only small amounts of dairy products at any one time (2-4oz/60-125ml).*

- *Eat dairy products in combination with other ingredients or foods.*

- *Eat dairy products, such as hard cheeses, that contain very little lactose.*

- *Use yogurt in food preparation. Yogurt contains high amounts of bacterial cultures that contain lactase.*

- *Add dry-milk powder to soups, casseroles, baking and so forth.*

- *Drink milk that is heated.*

- *Talk to a healthcare provider about the use of Lactaid or other commercially available lactase. Lactaid, when added to milk, breaks down the sugar and helps in the digestion of milk.*

Most dietitians will tell you to consume two to four servings of milk products daily. One cup (8oz/250ml) of milk or 1.75oz/50g of cheese equals about 320mg of calcium. If necessary, you may wish to increase your non-dairy options for calcium as well.

## CONSTIPATION AND GAS

If constipation or gas is an issue for you, eating more foods high in fiber, such as raw fruit, vegetables and bran, may help counteract the constipation. However, consistently eating large servings of foods very high in fiber will tend to decrease the absorption of calcium. Since fiber in the diet is good, try to take small amounts more frequently during the day. Use a food guide to know your fiber requirements and to gradually increase your fiber intake as needed. Magnesium is also known to decrease constipation (see Chapter 5). Most experts say constipation associated with a diet high in cheese is a myth, but be aware of the fat content of cheese if cholesterol is a concern.

Avoid the use of mineral oil as a laxative. Mineral oil decreases the absorption of fat soluble vitamins, including vitamin D which is necessary for the body to absorb its calcium.

**Tips:**

- *Drink water (six to eight glasses per day).*

- *Use natural laxatives, such as prune juice or figs.*

- *Eat fruits and vegetables high in roughage, such as apples, celery, corn, dried beans and peas.*

### FAT

Low-fat and high-fat foods are comparable in calcium content. If you want to decrease your fat intake, be selective about the foods you choose and look at the percentage of fat they contain. Low-fat dairy products are often a good choice.

**Tips:**

- *Avoid fried foods and cream sauces.*

- *If cholesterol is not an issue, hard cheeses are higher in calcium and, therefore, a good choice. Choose one percent cottage cheese over four percent cottage cheese. Choose foods that are low in fat, such as skim or one percent milk and low-fat yogurt.*

- *Eat a variety of fruits and vegetables. These are low in fat and are a good source of other necessary nutrients.*

## CALCIUM SUPPLEMENTS

Calcium is very important in childhood and adolescence, when the growing skeleton needs the most calcium for bone formation. We also need to be aware of our calcium intake as we get older. This is especially true for people who do not consume dairy products.

As we age, our dietary intake may change for any number of reasons: our taste buds are less sensitive; we may have fewer social engagements involving food; we have less interest in preparing a varied diet or preparing food in general. It is important to be aware of our nutritional needs.

Food remains the best source of calcium and dairy products are the easiest dietary source of calcium. Dairy products, such as milk, cheeses and yogurt, are an excellent source of calcium. Some foods, such as orange juice, cereals and breads, are fortified with calcium, but the calcium content of fortified foods varies.

As previously noted, research shows that individuals 50 years of age and over generally have a daily dietary intake of only 300mg to 700mg of calcium, which is less than the recommended 1,200mg per day. If you have tried to improve your calcium intake and still do not reach the recommended daily amount, then you may want to consider taking oral calcium supplements. While calcium is an important part of overall bone health, calcium alone will not prevent osteoporosis or restore lost bone. Be sure to discuss the value of supplements in preventing and treating osteoporosis with your doctor.

## Choosing a Supplement

Choose a supplement that meets your needs and preferences. Look on the label for the "elemental calcium" content. Elemental calcium is the actual amount of calcium in the supplement available for the body to absorb. In the United States and Canada, many labels with AUSP@ or a natural product number (NPN) do not indicate "elemental calcium." The amount of calcium noted on the label is the amount of elemental calcium. Read the label and note the amount of calcium supplementation you need in a day to meet your daily calcium requirement. If it is not clear to you, you may wish to check with your pharmacist before you buy the product.

### CALCIUM CONTENTS DIFFER

Calcium carbonate and calcium citrate are the forms of calcium that are best absorbed by the human body. Calcium carbonate contains a high percentage of elemental calcium (40 percent) and should be taken with a glass of water and with food to help to improve its breakdown and absorption. As food is digested, acid from the stomach helps to break down the calcium. Although calcium citrate has a lower percentage of elemental calcium (21 percent), it has a high bioavailability (ability to be absorbed) and can be taken on an empty stomach. Calcium citrate may be the best choice if you are on a proton pump inhibitor (Nexium or Prilosec for example).

Other forms of calcium, such as calcium phosphate, calcium lactate and calcium gluconate, are not as common, but are sometimes recommended.

Calcium phosphate at 38 percent elemental calcium is most commonly used in multivitamins and mineral supplements. It is not as well absorbed in the body as calcium carbonate and calcium citrate. Therefore, multivitamins alone may not provide enough calcium to meet your daily requirements.

Calcium lactate and calcium gluconate at 13 percent and nine percent elemental calcium respectively are both well absorbed in the body, but they have low amounts of elemental calcium. Consequently, you may need to take several doses to reach your daily required allotment.

Be sure to discuss these forms of calcium with your doctor, pharmacist or healthcare provider. Consider the advantages and disadvantages of each based on your own situation. The amount of calcium supplementation you need will be determined by a discussion with your doctor or registered dietitian, aided by the careful completion of your calcium intake chart.

Ask your doctor, registered dietitian or pharmacist about the best time to take calcium – with meals or on an empty stomach. Whatever the approach, it may be helpful to divide the total amount of calcium into two or three doses per day so that the body has smaller amounts to absorb at one time. However, that only works as long as you remember to take it two or three times a day! The most your body can absorb at one time is about 500mg of elemental calcium.

When choosing a supplement, be sure the product is:

- *Consistent and offers pure content. It is best to avoid calcium from oyster shells, dolomite or bone meal as they may contain toxic metals. In some brands of calcium supplements, the amount of calcium in each bottle may vary. Check the label to see that it has been assessed through a reliable source and meet certain standards. As noted earlier, the United States and Canada have instituted voluntary quality control standards for supplements.*

- *Easy to digest. To see if a particular calcium product is easily digested, place the calcium tablet in a small bowl of vinegar for 30 minutes. If the tablet dissolves within 30 minutes, it should easily dissolve in the stomach. Calcium supplements can be taken in several forms, including liquids, flavored chews, capsules and tablets (effervescent or chewable). Within these different forms are several types of calcium. Make sure to read the labels carefully.*

- *Easy to tolerate and convenient to take. As noted earlier in this chapter, some people have difficulty with gas or constipation. Try to increase your fluids and fiber or try a different type or brand of calcium. Start with a lower dose for a while and then increase it to your ideal dose. For some people, liquid or chewable preparations are easier to tolerate. Chewable forms are available as tablets or flavored chews. Some experts feel that calcium with magnesium preparations may lessen the constipation concern because the magnesium acts as a mild laxative. Talk with your pharmacist. You may have to try a few different brands and types of calcium to find the best one for you. Be sure to choose a preparation that is convenient to take and fits within your budget, otherwise you may not take it as often as you should.*

- *Adequately absorbed. Calcium supplements may deliver a different amount of elemental calcium per gram of the calcium type. It is the amount of elemental calcium that you want to increase, but any amount greater than 500mg of elemental calcium at one time will not be absorbed by the body.*

You may not need the more expensive designer products that offer a combination of vitamins and minerals, such as magnesium, phosphorus and vitamins D and K. With the exception of vitamin D, most experts feel these vitamins and minerals can be adequately obtained through a well-balanced diet. If you do take a combination, be sure to know the amount of each product in the preparation. Combination products rarely have the right amounts of all the vitamins and minerals you, as an individual, need.

There are many different calcium preparations, so talk with your doctor, registered dietitian or pharmacist about the different preparations and which one is best for you.

## Quality Control

**In the United States, look for AUSP@ on the label. AUSP@, which was established by the United States Pharmacopeia, signifies that a product has met voluntary quality standards of purity and dissolution. In Canada, look for a Natural Product Number (NPN). NPN will be noted on the front of the label followed by a number. NPN replaces the DIN (Drug Identification Number), which also represented a quality controlled product.**

### CALCIUM INTERACTS WITH SOME MEDICATIONS

Check with your doctor or pharmacist about when to take other medications in relation to the calcium you choose. Calcium will bind to bisphosphonates. Some doctors suggest avoiding dietary calcium and supplements the night before and the day you take your morning oral dose of bisphosphonate. For example, etidronate (Didrocal), alendronate (Fosamax) and risedronate (Actonel) should not be taken at the same time of day as calcium, either as foods or supplements. These medications are discussed in Chapter 11.

Calcium has been shown to interfere with the absorption of iron supplements, thyroid medication and the antibiotic tetracycline. Be sure that your doctor and pharmacist are aware of all medications and supplements you are taking. Even over-the-counter medications and herbal remedies can cause possible drug interactions.

### COMPARE THE COSTS AND EFFICACY OF CALCIUM

Compare price of calcium supplements, but be sure to buy an effective product. Talk with your pharmacist about the differences in absorption and the costs of the products. Some insurance plans and healthcare programs may pay for therapeutic calcium supplements. Ask your doctor or insurance agent if reimbursement for the cost of the calcium is possible.

### COMMON CALCIUM SUPPLEMENTS

Calcium carbonate preparations include Tums 200mg to 400mg, Calcite 500mg, Calsan chewable 500mg, Caltrate 600mg, Os-Cal 250mg to 600mg. Be cautious about using products claiming to be "bone builders." They may include vitamin D or magnesium, but you can get adequate vitamin D and magnesium through other types of supplements or a well-balanced diet. Calcium is calcium – ensure you get the amount of calcium your body needs by talking with your doctor or healthcare provider.

### SIDE EFFECTS OF CALCIUM SUPPLEMENTS

If you have a history of kidney stones, you may be at an increased risk of recurrence. In such cases, do not take calcium supplements unless directed and supervised by a doctor. Sometimes the presence of kidney stones, which contain calcium oxalates, can be a clue to an underlying cause of osteoporosis. If you need to take a calcium supplement, your doctor might suggest taking calcium citrate and encourage you to drink lots of fluids.

## CHAPTER 4 KEY POINTS

- Recommended daily calcium intake for adults over 50 is 1,000mg to 1,200mg, including both dietary and supplemental.

- One 8oz/250ml glass of cow or soy milk (fortified) has about 320mg of calcium.

- The calcium you get from the food you eat is best.

- There are many easy ways to increase your dietary calcium such as substituting cow's or soy milk for water when cooking or adding cheese, soy beans or other kinds of beans to a recipe.

- Calculate your daily calcium intake at least once a year and compare to recommended daily calcium intake.

- Too much calcium may be harmful.

- Calcium alone cannot prevent osteoporosis or restore bone health.

- If you do not meet the recommended calcium intake through diet alone, adjust your diet or add a calcium supplement.

- There are many options for calcium supplements if you need one. Choose one that suits you best.

# CHAPTER 5

# Vitamin D and Other Vitamins and Minerals

Most experts recommend that adults under 50 need 400IU to 1,000IU of vitamin D supplementation per day and those over 50 need about 800IU to 2,000IU supplementation per day. As medical guidelines are updated, experts are suggesting up to 2,000IU of calcium intake per day is safe. Intakes of 4,000IU to 5,000IU per day may be safe, but can be associated with possible kidney stones, which are very painful

The benefits of vitamin D appear to reach beyond the skeleton. Research is being done on the impact of vitamin D on common cancers, autoimmune disorders, infections, cardiovascular disease and muscle strength. For our purposes, we will discuss the vitamin D group, the need for vitamin D, its sources and the optimal levels for bone health. We will also review other vitamins and minerals that contribute to healthy bones.

## VITAMIN D

Vitamin D is essential in calcium and phosphorus metabolism and required for normal development of bones and teeth. It is a fat-soluble vitamin that when ingested or produced by the skin is changed in the liver and kidney to its active form, known as calcitriol (1, 25, hydroxy-vitamin D). Other forms include vitamin D2 (ergocalciferol, a plant source) and vitamin D3 (cholecalciferol, an animal source).

Known as the sunshine vitamin, vitamin D is an important part of bone health, both in the prevention and treatment of osteoporosis. For many years, we have known the value of vitamin D in the normal development and maintenance of strong bones and teeth. The role of vitamin D in nerve and muscle tissue is now showing its value in fall and fracture prevention. Studies have shown that, for people over 65, high vitamin D levels can improve walking compared to people with low vitamin D levels. Studies pooled together (called a meta-analysis) show that, among older individuals who take a vitamin D supplement at a dose of 700IU to 1,000IU per day, the risk of falling is reduced by nearly 20 percent.

Research continues to point out that many people are still deficient in vitamin D. Between 40 and 100 percent of elderly men and women living in an institution, such as a care home or hospital, are deficient in vitamin D and more than 50 percent of women already taking medication to treat osteoporosis are also deficient in vitamin D.

## VITAMIN D SOURCES

Vitamin D comes from two main sources: dietary intake and the skin's exposure to the sun.

### Dietary Sources

Few foods naturally contain or are fortified with vitamin D. Natural food sources of vitamin D include fatty fish, fish liver oils and egg yolks. Foods fortified with vitamin D include margarine, milk, orange juice, cheese, butter and yogurt. Check the food label for actual vitamin D content.

| Food | Serving | Estimated Vitamin D |
|---|---|---|
| Fresh wild salmon | 3.5oz/100g | 750IU |
| Canned salmon | 3.5oz/100g | 450IU |
| Canned mackerel or sardines | 3.5oz /100g | 360IU |
| Fresh farmed salmon | 3.5oz/100g | 200IU |
| Canned tuna in oil | 3.5oz/100g | 200IU |
| Margarine | 1 tbsp/15ml | 90IU |
| Milk, fortified or enriched soy or rice beverage | 1 cup/250ml | 90IU |
| Egg yolk | 1 | 20IU |

# Sunshine

When the sun's rays hit the skin, vitamin D is produced. Sunshine is considered the best, most efficient source for your daily requirement of vitamin D. Research shows that when using simulated sunlight, a single minimal erythemal (red) skin dose will raise circulating levels of vitamin D [1, 25(OH)D] comparable to ingestion of 10,000IU to 25,000IU of vitamin D3. Exposure to between five and 10 minutes of sunlight can provide the equivalent of about 3,000IU of vitamin D.

Getting adequate amounts of vitamin D may be difficult for people living near or north of the forty-second parallel. In North America, the forty-second parallel runs roughly from New York State on the east coast to Washington State on the west coast. Therefore, people living in the northern United States and Canada need to supplement their vitamin D intake from October through March to compensate for the lack of sun exposure on the skin, specifically the ultraviolet B (UVB) rays. The amount of vitamin D you receive from your skin's exposure to UVB rays decreases due to any of the following:

- *Age. The skin of older adults often cannot synthesize vitamin D as efficiently and their kidneys are less able to convert vitamin D to its active hormone form.*

- *Dark skin. The amount of melanin or pigment in your skin can decrease absorption.*

- *Amount of smog in the air or use of sunscreen can filter the UVB rays.*

- *Cloud cover or time spent in the shade can reduce UVB ray exposure by half.*

- *Living north of forty-second parallel. UVB from the sun in northern regions, especially in fall and winter, is less useful.*

- *Time of day. UVB rays tend to be weakest outside the peak hours of 10 a.m. and 3 p.m.*

- *Wearing long robes or head coverings or staying indoors.*

> Daily sunshine exposure of 15 to 30 minutes with maximum skin exposure and no sunscreen should provide your daily recommended dose of vitamin D.

Given concerns about skin cancer caused by to too much exposure to the sun, some dermatologists suggest limiting sun exposure or using a sunscreen lotion with a high sun protection factor (SPF). It is important to assess and consider your personal sun exposure, cancer risk and vitamin D intake.

The amount of sun exposure you need in any one day to get your recommended dose of vitamin D depends on various factors as outlined above. Experts agree, however, that sun exposure of about ten to thirty minutes a day will probably provide the required daily dose of vitamin D. Adjust the time to consider the different factors mentioned above, and remember, excessive exposure to the sun may increase the risk of skin cancer and wrinkling or drying of the skin.

## HOW MUCH VITAMIN D DO I NEED?

The recommended dosage of vitamin D for people over 50 is 800IU to 2,000IU per day. Research is underway to assess daily requirements that may well exceed these amounts. Many experts feel the current tolerable upper limit of daily vitamin D intake for adults over age 50 is 2,000IU, while some experts say 2,500IU per day is the upper limit. Some individuals take as much as 5,000IU per day, but these levels might result in high levels of calcium in the blood and urine and may result in kidney stones. Talk with your doctor about the latest research and your needs.

Vitamin D levels can be easily checked by your doctor if there is a concern about malabsorption of this vitamin. Most specialists do not check vitamin D levels routinely prior to starting vitamin D supplements. Some experts suggest that if you are going to measure the levels, the best time is three months after you start on a vitamin D supplement. Other experts feel you should only measure vitamin D levels if you are on treatment and still losing bone or experiencing fractures. Discuss with your doctor whether you should have your level checked or just go on a good amount of vitamin D. If you miss a dose and later remember, it is safe to double the dose to make up for it. If diagnosed with vitamin D deficiency, some doctors may suggest a large loading dose of 50,000IU per day or weekly of vitamin D2 (Ostoforte) for a short period of time.

Vitamin D supplements may be either vitamin D2 or D3, which are similar. Vitamin D3 is the naturally-occurring form of vitamin D and thought to be more than three times as effective as the same amount of vitamin D2 in affecting blood levels and maintaining those levels longer.

When taking a non-prescription supplement, the vitamin D3 form, rather than the vitamin D2 form, is generally used. Vitamin D2 is sometimes used in multivitamin preparations. Vitamin D2 may also be written as a prescription for 50,000IU of vitamin D2 ergocalciferol. While this may seem like a strong dose, remember, vitamin D2 is less potent than vitamin D3. Most supplements now consist of vitamin D3 rather than vitamin D2. Vitamin D2 may be appropriate for vegans or anyone who avoids animal products. It is derived from a plant source, whereas D3 is manufactured from an animal source. Check with your pharmacist to ensure it is the right supplement for you.

Calcitriol is the active form of vitamin D, which is infrequently used and more expensive than vitamins D2 or D3. Some studies with calcitriol have demonstrated significant decrease in fractures of the spine among individuals with severe osteoporosis. However, calcitriol can do its job too well and help absorb too much calcium. With too much vitamin D, calcium levels can build up in the blood and settle in parts of the body where it should not, and thus cause damage. This could cause calcium kidney stones, which can be painful and may damage the kidney. Calcitriol treatment should only be prescribed by doctors with expertise in treating patients with osteoporosis.

# OTHER VITAMINS AND MINERALS

## Vitamin A

Vitamin A is a fat-soluble vitamin essential for normal growth and development of the teeth, bones and the tissues that form the skin and line the body cavities. It also helps the body resist infection and provides nutrition to parts of the eye. Too much vitamin A may be bad for your body. Excess vitamin A can actually cause bone loss.

Smokers who supplement their diet with beta-carotene, which is found in dark green and orange-yellow vegetables and converted in the body to vitamin A, increase their risk of lung cancer. Excessive consumption of retinol supplements, such as vitamin A and beta-carotene, especially in the elderly, can produce vitamin A toxicity, which may have acute or chronic effects. Check with your doctor or pharmacist if these concerns apply to your medical situation.

Cod liver oil used regularly as a supplement is somewhat controversial. While granny may have suggested a spoonful a day, granny may have been wrong on this one. Cod liver oil contains both vitamin D and a very high level of vitamin A, which if taken in excess could exceed the daily maximum requirement and result in toxicity. If you are taking cod liver oil, be sure that the total dose of vitamin A is less than 5,000IU per day or you may be making the problem worse.

### DIETARY SOURCES OF VITAMIN A

Vitamin A that is converted from its precursor (or carotenoids) comes from both animal sources as retinol and plant sources as beta-carotene. Animal sources of vitamin A, such as liver, eggs and milk, are absorbed in a very usable and active form. The precursor is the fat-soluble pigment found naturally in fruits and vegetables and acts as an antioxidant. It resembles carotene which is one of several yellow, red, orange or green antioxidant compounds found in dark green and yellow vegetables and some fruits, such as tomatoes, apricots, oranges, cantaloupes, prunes and pineapples.

Vitamin A activity in foods is expressed as retinol equivalents (RE), the resulting amount of retinol after conversion in the body. One ingested retinol equivalent is equal to 6mg of beta-carotene, which is one of the active forms of vitamin A stored in the body, primarily in the liver and the adipose tissue or body fat. The suggested daily requirement for adults is about 1,000mg. Because vitamin A has much greater toxic potential in larger doses, beta-carotene, an organic compound with a lower concentration of vitamin A, is a safer food supplement than a pure vitamin A supplement.

Research has found that high daily intake of supplemental retinol vitamin A (greater than 2,000IU per day) affects bone remodeling and can be associated with an increased risk of hip fractures. There is no similar evidence between beta-carotene vitamin A intake and hip fractures or increased risk of osteoporosis.

The daily requirement of vitamin A for post-menopausal women is about 2,500IU or less; men is similar. Younger menstruating women require a little more vitamin A per day, but less than 5,000IU.

## Vitamin K

Vitamin K is a fat-soluble vitamin that has an important role in blood clotting. It has another role in bone metabolism and is a potential protector against osteoporosis. Further research is needed to determine the appropriate vitamin K intake and the impact of anticoagulant (blood thinning) therapy on bone health.

People who form blood clots too easily or too quickly and may be on a drug such as Warfarin (Coumadin) should talk with their healthcare provider. Warfarin can work to decrease the activity of vitamin K and lengthen the time it takes for a clot to form. However, this anticoagulant may also negatively affect your bone health. If this is your situation, know your vitamin K intake and keep it consistent from day to day. Work with your healthcare provider to best manage your treatment and protect your bone health.

## DIETARY SOURCES OF VITAMIN K

As with most dietary vitamins, vitamin K is obtained through a varied and well-balanced diet. Vitamin K is found in dark green and leafy vegetables, alfalfa, oats, wheat and rye. The average suggested daily requirement of vitamin K is about 90mcg (micrograms) per day for women and 120mcg for men. Just one-half cup/125ml of broccoli can offer more than twice the daily requirement.

## Phosphorus

Phosphorus is an important mineral that requires vitamin D for its absorption and metabolism. It is an essential element of bone formation and has many other functions such as cell growth, carbohydrate metabolism, protein syntheses, and muscle and kidney function. Normally excreted by the kidneys and intestines, an excessive amount of phosphorus in the body is rare, but an excess of phosphorus can interfere with calcium uptake. Any excess phosphorus would likely be due to renal or kidney disease or over supplementation.

### DIETARY SOURCES OF PHOSPHORUS

A healthy diet has enough phosphorus-containing foods to meet the roughly 800mg per day suggested requirement. High protein foods, such as milk products, eggs, meats, poultry and fresh or canned fish are the best source of phosphorus. Almonds, string beans, carrots, raisins and cucumbers are other good sources.

## Magnesium

Magnesium is a mineral needed by most cells in the body. Magnesium helps to move nutrients in and out of cells and maintain normal muscle. It also serves important functions related to nerves and bones as well as many other body systems.

### DIETARY SOURCES

Most experts feel you can achieve the recommended 200mg to 400mg per day of magnesium through a well-balanced, healthy diet provided you absorb the nutrients. Good sources of magnesium are some fish, nuts, vegetables, fruits and whole grains.

| Food | Serving | Estimated Magnesium |
|------|---------|---------------------|
| Halibut | 3oz/84g | 90mg |
| Dry roasted almonds or cashews | 1oz/28g | 80mg |
| Frozen or cooked spinach | 0.5 cup/125m | 80mg |
| Yogurt or skim milk | 1 cup/250ml | 45mg |
| Brown rice | 0.5 cup/125m | 40mg |
| Whole grain bread | single slice | 25mg |

A little secret for chocolate lovers – chocolate that is high in cocoa is an excellent source of magnesium.

## ALKALINE (BASIC) OR ACID-PRODUCING FOODS AND BONE HEALTH

The impact of alkaline and acid-producing foods on bone health is subject to debate. There is some suggestion that alkali-forming foods, such as fruits and vegetables, might be advantageous for bone health. We certainly know that there is good evidence that diet can have a favorable effect on cholesterol and cardiovascular disease, so this is one more reason to eat a healthy, well-balanced diet. More research will help to clarify the issues.

# CHAPTER 5 KEY POINTS

- Vitamin D is necessary for the absorption of calcium and prevention of osteoporosis.

- Many people are deficient in vitamin D.

- Recommended daily intake for adults over 50 ranges from 800IU to 2,000IU of vitamin D.

- Few foods naturally provide enough vitamin D.

- Some foods are fortified with vitamin D. Check the package label.

- Daily sunshine exposure of 15 to 30 minutes with maximum skin exposure and no sunscreen should provide your daily recommended dose of vitamin D.

- Vitamin A, K and phosphorus are all important for bone metabolism, but should be provided in adequate amounts in a healthy, well-balanced diet.

- Vitamin A supplementation may increase health risks if taken in excess.

## CHAPTER 6

# The Importance of Exercising and Safe Movement

**It is important to consult with a doctor or physical therapist before commencing or adjusting any exercise program.**

---

The importance of physical activity on bone health is well recognized. Studies show that a person who is inactive or immobilized for a period of time will lose bone. For example, an astronaut in space, weightless (non-weight-bearing) for several weeks, will show muscle wasting, a decrease in strength, a significant calcium loss and a decrease in bone density. Similar muscle wasting and bone loss is seen when a cast is worn for several weeks. While most of us will not spend time in space, immobility from lower extremity fractures or surgery is common.

Research also shows that weight-bearing exercises reduce the risk of osteoporosis. Exercise is an effective approach to bone health because the bone responds to weight-bearing activities by increasing in strength. Studies show that physically active people have higher bone density in their lumbar spine and hips than people of the same sex, age and height who are inactive. Activities such as walking, dancing, climbing stairs and cross-country skiing may all help to maintain or improve your bone density.

Physical activity is either non weight-bearing, such as swimming, or weight-bearing, such as walking.

## NON WEIGHT-BEARING ACTIVITIES

During non weight-bearing activities, the muscles contract and pull and apply stress indirectly to the bone. This stress on the bone promotes bone formation and a healthy skeleton. An example of this formation through non weight-bearing exercise is the baseball pitcher's throwing arm. The bone strength is increased from the stress that muscle places on the bone from the activity of throwing a ball. These exercises are also referred to as weight-resistant or strength training exercises. Examples include working with free weights, weight-training machines or exercise bands.

## WEIGHT-BEARING ACTIVITIES

During weight-bearing activities, weight is transmitted through the bone. This promotes bone formation and a healthy skeleton. When specifically trying to increase bone density, weight-bearing activities are preferred over non-weight-bearing activities as they are more valuable for muscle strengthening, balance and improved bone health.

The type of exercise you choose should match your current health status. If you have or are at risk of developing osteoporosis, then a well-regulated, weight-bearing exercise program would be the most beneficial for you.

Problems with the heart, lungs, joints or other pre-existing conditions may prevent you from doing certain exercises. Check with your doctor before starting any exercise program that may aggravate an existing problem. People with arthritis may find some weight-bearing exercises inappropriate. Exercising in water may be a creative solution.

Work with a doctor or a physical therapist who is experienced with osteoporosis to ensure you choose a program that is right for your body and health status. If you have not been exercising for a while, start out cautiously. As you improve your endurance, slowly increase the number of repetitions of an exercise and eventually increase the variety of exercises you can do. Exercise programs should include stretching, muscle-strengthening and balance exercises appropriate for you.

## WALK, WALK, WALK

Our focus for exercise and bone health is to build stronger bones and improve strength and balance to prevent falls. Some experts believe walking is the best activity for getting in shape and maintaining better bone health.

*Walking is fundamental to good bone health. There is no downside to walking if done safely.*

Walking has a number of health benefits. It provides cardio exercise that improves the heart and consumes calories to fight obesity and diabetes. Walking improves mental health, reduces depression, increases self-esteem and improves your quality of sleep. Muscle tone, strength and stamina will improve and result in better balance and decrease your risk of falls.

Walking benefits people of all ages. As a regular physical activity, walking is inexpensive and you can walk almost anywhere. Walking is a wonderful social and family activity. It helps to reduce anxiety and tension and can be an up-lifting, relaxing and meditative opportunity in the midst of a crazy or bad day. Some community groups use walking as a social or educational activity. Walking is a healthy activity that can be shared by all generations.

As with any activity, you want to be safe while you walk. Check with your doctor or a fitness instructor to determine if you have any limitations that might prevent you from walking safely (see Get up and Go Test in the Glossary). Discuss the need for a balance and gait assessment with your doctor or healthcare team. Consider whether your balance, vision, hearing or joints are impaired or compromised. By talking with a physical or occupational therapist, you may find ways to minimize these issues and improve your walking.

Begin your walking program slowly. Do not overdo it or you may not want to continue. Talk with your doctor to determine how far you can comfortably walk without becoming tired. Fifteen to 30 minutes is generally a good start. Plan a weekly schedule of at least three times per week. For a cardiovascular benefit, you may need a minimum of three times per week for at least 30 minutes each time. Some experts suggest doing cardio exercises five to six times a week and combine these cardio exercises with weight training three times a week. Beginners are encouraged to walk shorter distances five times weekly at first. You should not feel any discomfort or stiffness after the first week. Build up to your optimum level.

Always make sure you are safe in the environment where you walk. Walking areas should be well lit so you can see any obstacles. Wear good supportive shoes and be sure that you are stable on your feet. Use mobility aids, if necessary, to keep your balance and hip protectors as an extra safety measure. You want to feel steady, safe and secure as you walk (see Chapter 10 for more details).

The descriptions of the exercises in this book pertain to the prevention and treatment of osteoporosis. If you want a total body workout, you will have to add other exercises to your regime. If you plan to join a community or private fitness program, try to find a program with an instructor certified in the field of seniors or bone and joint health.

## JOINING A FITNESS PROGRAM

One option for a regular fitness routine is to join a community fitness program. These programs can vary in training and safety. Many organizations offer specialty programs specific to bone and joint health. Talk with your local osteoporosis groups to see which fitness programs are recommended. Use the following questions as a guide to compare fitness programs and finding the one that's right for you.

- *Are the instructors certified to lead classes for your age group, disease state or condition?*

- *Do the instructors pace the class for the participants?*

- *Are you encouraged to go at your own speed and compete only with yourself?*

- *Do the instructors answer questions satisfactorily?*

- *Is there a warm-up and cool-down phase?*

- *Does each workout include stretching?*

Do not rely solely on the instructor's knowledge. Speak with your doctor, physical therapist or healthcare provider before starting an exercise program of any kind. It is never too late to start exercising. Work with your doctor or healthcare provider to find the right exercise program. It is important to find a qualified instructor who can help you develop good habits for movement, increasing your strength and balance, and avoiding postures or movements that can lead to injury during normal activities.

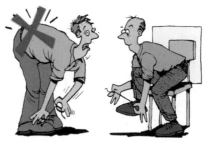

Without strong muscles and bones, simple everyday tasks can cause a fracture of a bone like the spine

## EXERCISE CONSIDERATIONS

## Be Safe

Since there are varying degrees of osteoporosis, be sure you know your own risk of osteoporosis and fracture before beginning any exercise program. Be sure you have an instructor qualified in bone health and exercise. Remember to move gently. If you are at high risk of osteoporosis, avoid jarring and impact activities. Be aware of your movement and how it impacts your bones. Learn how to bend and lift correctly. If in doubt about an exercise, check it out with an exercise specialist. If you experience pain or discomfort when doing an exercise, stop the exercise immediately and speak with your healthcare provider.

No exercise is safe if you injure yourself while doing it. Be careful.

## Plan Ahead

Commit to a time of day to exercise. Make it a priority – the benefits of exercise outweigh the inconvenience. A suitable routine should include exercising about 15 minutes twice a day, three to four times a week. Keep a record of your progress by recording how you feel after each workout. To keep it interesting and to work different muscles, choose a few different exercises each week.

By exercising at the same time each day or days of the week, you will develop a routine that will become easier to follow over time. If you exercise "when I get around to it," you probably won't get around to it. If you don't have a plan, it won't happen despite your best intentions.

## Breathe

Muscles require oxygen to work. Regular, rhythmical breathing as you exercise will help to reduce the internal pressure in your body and allow oxygen to get to the body tissues as it should. During an exercise, breathe out during the exertion phase and breathe in as you relax. Breathe deeply from your diaphragm. Place your hands on your lower ribs and feel them expand and contract as you breathe.

## Repetitions

After repeating each exercise three times, remember to completely relax. Relaxing between exercises allows your muscles to gain the full benefit of the exercise. Slowly increase the number of repetitions. If your doctor agrees, try adding one repetition per day to a maximum of 10 repetitions.

## Posture

Correct posture for a naturally fit person is when the chin is pulled in, the person is standing tall and erect, and the shoulders are pulled back. The lower back is arched backward and the abdominal muscles are pulled in to support the lower back.

Strong abdominal muscles will support the spine and help with correct posture. By maintaining correct posture, you will avoid putting undue stress on your spine. A correct posture will also help promote deeper, easier breathing and more efficient food digestion. Correct posture, whether sitting, standing or lying down, is important if the muscles and the entire body are to function properly.

## CHAPTER 6 KEY POINTS

- **Exercise is good for the whole body.**
- **The focus for exercise and bone health is to build stronger bones and improve strength and balance to prevent falls and fractures.**
- **The type and amount of exercise you choose should match your health status. Talk with your doctor to determine your health status.**
- **Walking is fundamental to good bone health.**
- **Walking 15 to 30 minutes three times a week is generally a good start to an exercise program.**
- **Plan ahead and make regular exercise a priority.**
- **Weight-bearing, strengthening and balance exercises help to reduce the risk of osteoporosis and falls.**
- **When exercising, consider the benefits of safe movements, breathing, number of repetitions and proper posture.**
- **If you join a group, be sure the instructor is properly certified in working with osteoporosis or older adults.**

# CHAPTER 7
# Exercises

## CHOOSING THE APPROPRIATE EXERCISES

It is important to work with your doctor, physical therapist or healthcare provider to find the right exercise program for you. Your program should take into account your health status and fracture risk. Your fracture risk is generally based on your bone mineral density and your 10-year risk of fracture test results along with your osteoporosis and fracture risk assessments. These are outlined in Part 3 of this book.

Based on your current health status, identify the group below that best describes your situation.

**Group 1 – individuals at low risk of fracture.** If you are healthy, at low risk of developing osteoporosis or fracturing a bone, choose a fitness program that offers exercises that have the most desirable effect on bone.

**Group 2 – individuals at moderate risk of fracture.** If you are at moderate risk of developing osteoporosis or fracturing a bone, start a prevention program with the appropriate weight-bearing exercises in consultation with your doctor or physical therapist.

**Group 3 – individuals at high risk of fracture.** If you have been diagnosed with osteoporosis or have had a low-trauma fracture, work with a doctor or physical therapist to determine which movements and exercises are appropriate and safe.

After you have identified your risk level for fracture, work with your healthcare provider to chart your course.

## CHARTING YOUR COURSE

The exercises in this book are presented as:

- *Set A – Stretching exercises*

- *Set B – Balance exercises*

Use the Exercise Chart below to complete the "Exercise" and "Repetitions Planned" in consultation with your physical therapist or doctor. Choose three exercises from each set of exercises. Next, choose the number of repetitions that will benefit you the most given your age, gender and medical history. Then, with your doctor or physical therapist, finish filling out the Exercise Chart. Follow the exercises as described. As you exercise, fill in the chart. Completing the chart is an important step in your exercise routine as it will map your progress. Download this Exercise Chart at osteoporosisbook.com

## Exercise Chart

| Date | Exercise | Repetitions Planned | Repetitions Completed | Time Spent (minutes) |
|------|----------|---------------------|-----------------------|----------------------|
|      |          |                     |                       |                      |
|      |          |                     |                       |                      |
|      |          |                     |                       |                      |
|      |          |                     |                       |                      |
|      |          |                     |                       |                      |
|      |          |                     |                       |                      |
|      |          |                     |                       |                      |
|      |          |                     |                       |                      |
|      |          |                     |                       |                      |
|      |          |                     |                       |                      |

## LET'S START EXERCISING

- Read and follow the description of each exercise.
- Keep your body aligned.
- Keep your eyes looking forward.

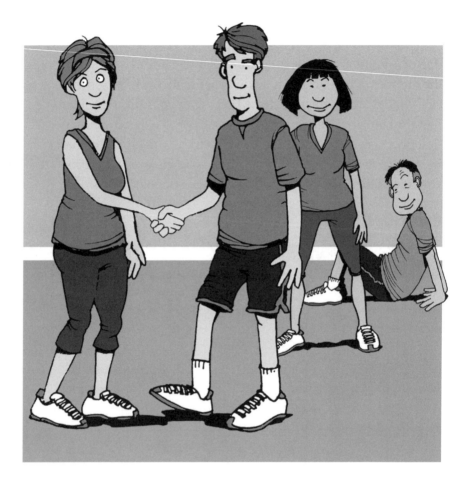

Regular daily exercise is good for not only your heart and lungs, but also your muscles and bones. Muscle conditioning, such as strengthening, provides additional insurance against falling because of poor balance or reduced flexibility. If done improperly, they could result in injury. When done properly, these exercises are designed to be beneficial in strengthening weak muscles and stretching tight muscles. If you have severe kyphosis, talk with a physical therapist or exercise specialist before undertaking these exercises.

**The exercises in this book should not cause any pain or discomfort. If you feel pain or discomfort, stop the exercise and omit it from your program until you talk with your doctor or physical therapist.**

Arm movements in these exercises are used to gain thoracic spinal extension. Lift your arms above your shoulder height (extension) slowly and cautiously, feel the stretch and do not go past the point of comfort. If there is any pain associated with this movement, avoid the movement and discuss the pain with your doctor or physical therapist.

If you find the exercises in this book too easy or mild, you might want to contact your local or national osteoporosis organization to find an appropriate osteoporosis exercise program in your community.

## SET A: STRETCHING EXERCISES

Stretching exercises are an important part of any exercise routine. These exercises will help to relax tight muscles in order to get the most benefit out of the Set B exercises.

## 1. Body Contraction

Lie on your back with your legs straight and your arms straight by your sides. Breathe normally; tighten your arms, back, stomach, seat and thigh muscles. At the same time, press your arms and knees into the floor. Hold for a count of three and relax. Do not hold your breath.

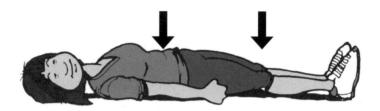

## 2. Back of leg stretch

Lie on your back with your head straight, your eyes looking up and your legs straight. Pull your toes up toward your head. Slowly push the back of your knees into the floor as you tighten your thigh muscles and try to lift only your heels off the floor. Hold for a count of 15, relax and repeat.

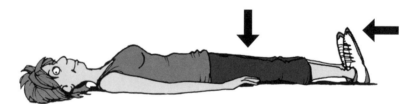

## 3. Pelvic Stabilizer

**Use your abdominal muscles, not your seat or buttock muscles.**

Lie on your back. With knees bent, tighten your tummy muscles and feel your lower back flatten onto the floor. The buttocks should not come off the floor. Hold for a count of three and relax.

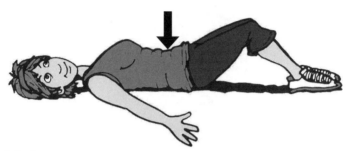

## 4. Bridging
**Keep your tummy pulled in tight.**

Lie on your back with your knees bent. Lift your stomach, hips and thighs off the floor. Hold for a count of three, relax and repeat.

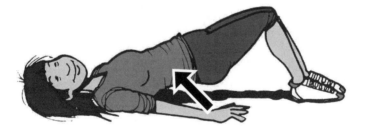

## 5. Inner thigh stretch

Lie on your back. Bend both knees. Pull your tummy in. Keeping your knees bent and both hips on the floor, slowly lower your left leg away from your body. Feel the stretch on your inner thigh. Hold for a count of 15 and return your leg to the center. Repeat with your right leg.

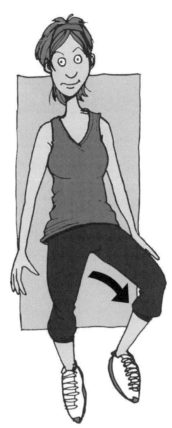

## 6. Knee to Chest

**Keep your spine straight, your lower back flat on the floor, your tummy pulled in tight and your eyes looking up.**

Lie on your back. Bend both knees and keep your feet on the floor. Lift your left knee up as close to your chest as possible. Grasp your left knee and gently pull it a little closer to your chest. Hold for a count of three. Slowly lower your leg, keeping your knee bent so that your foot ends up on the floor with your knee still bent. Repeat with your right leg.

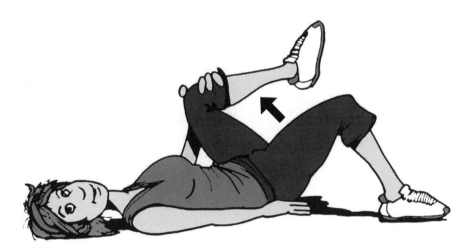

## 7. Knees to Chest

**Keep your spine straight, your lower back flat on the floor, your tummy pulled in tight and your eyes looking up.**

Lie on your back. Lift your left leg close to your chest and lift your right leg level with your left leg. Grasp both knees and pull them toward your shoulders. Hold for a count of three, then slowly relax your arms; keep both knees bent and lower your feet to the floor. If you cannot keep your back flat on the floor, you need to talk to your doctor or physical therapist for an easier lower abdominal exercise.

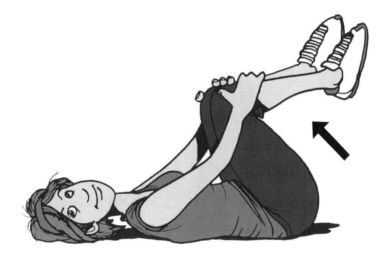

## 8. Knee Push

Lie flat on your back with your legs straight, keeping your abdominal muscles contracted. Bend your right knee above your right hip and place both hands on your knee. As you count to 15, push your knee against your hands and your hands against your knee. Relax and repeat with your left knee.

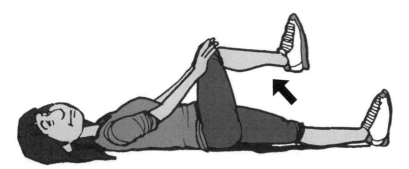

## 9. Knee Extension

**Keep your tummy pulled in tight and your lower back flat against the floor and eyes looking up. Do not do this exercise if you have lower back or hip pain.**

Start by lying on the floor with both your knees bent. Lift your left foot so that your left leg is straight (about 45 degrees above the floor) and hold. Then, bending your knee slowly, lower your left foot to the floor. Repeat with your right leg.

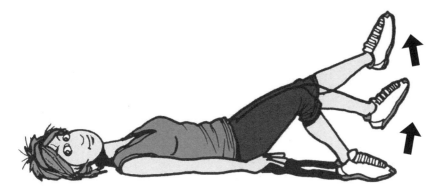

## 10. Leg Slide

**Keep your leg in contact with the floor as you slide it out to the side.**

Start by lying on the floor with both knees bent. Pull your tummy in tight. Straighten your left leg on the floor. Slowly slide your left leg out to the side away from your body as far as you comfortably can. Lead with your left heel and keep the toes pointed to the ceiling. Return your left leg to the middle and repeat with the other leg.

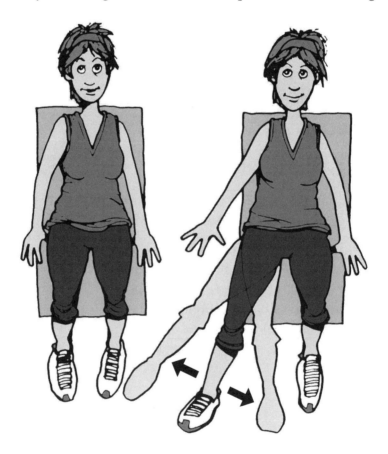

## 11. Knees to side

**Keep both feet flat on the floor at all times.**

Lie flat on the floor with knees bent. Keeping both shoulders touching the floor and your knees together, slowly and gently lower both legs to the left. Try to touch the floor, count to three, and then bring them back to the center. Repeat by lowering both legs to the right side.

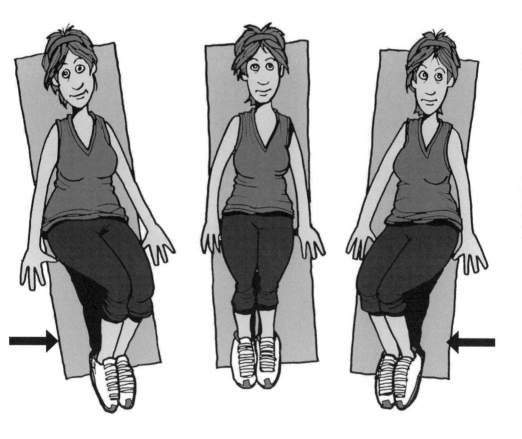

## 12. Leg Roll

Lie on your back with both legs straight. Bend your left ankle and point that foot to the ceiling. Slowly roll that foot and leg away from the body so that the toes touch the floor. Then, roll your foot back up so that your toes are again pointing to the ceiling. Roll your left foot and leg in towards the right leg so that the toes touch the floor. Then, roll your foot back up, so that your toes are pointing to the ceiling. Repeat with your right leg.

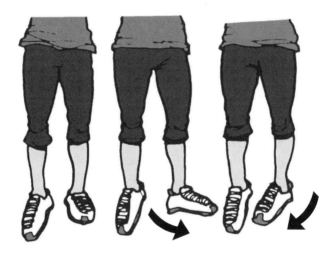

## 13. Arm Stretch

**Do not lift your arms above shoulder height if you have severe kyphosis or if it causes pain in your shoulders or back.**

Starting with arms at your sides, lead with your thumb and slowly raise your straight left arm above your head. Lower your arm behind your head to touch the floor. Repeat with your right arm.

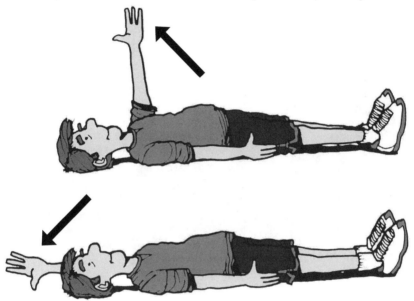

## 14. Double Elbow Press

Lie on your back. Slide your upper arms away from your sides and up to shoulder height. Bend your elbows so that your hands point to the ceiling. Slowly press your upper arms, elbows and back of head into the floor (at right angles to the floor). Hold for a count of 15, relax and repeat.

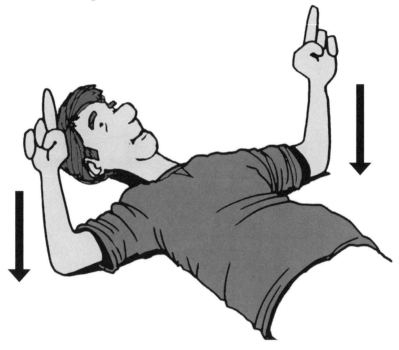

## 15. Long Stretch on Your Stomach

**Keep your chin tucked in. A pillow under your stomach may help you feel more comfortable. If you have severe kyphosis, you may need to place an additional pillow or two under your abdomen when lying face down.**

Lie on your stomach. Straighten your legs and keep them together. Point your toes away from you as far as possible while tightening your stomach and seat muscles. Slide your arms around to stretch out in front of your head. Stretch as if you were being pulled from your wrists and toes at the same time. Hold for a count of 15, relax and repeat.

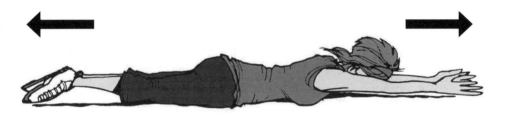

## 16. Extension of All Four Limbs

**Be cautious if you have severe kyphosis. As you stretch, do not go past your point of comfort.**

A.  Lie flat on your stomach with your legs straight and your arms by your sides. A small pillow under your forehead and/or stomach may make you more comfortable. Slide your left arm above your head and straighten it. Raise it off the floor as high as is comfortable. Relax. Repeat with your right arm. Repeat the entire exercise.

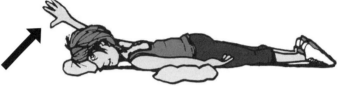

B.  Slowly tighten the muscle above your left knee (quadriceps), lift your left leg from the hip and hold for three seconds. Relax. Repeat with your right leg. Repeat the entire exercise.

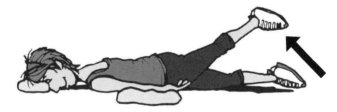

C.  With your left arm straight above your head, slowly raise your left arm and your right leg at the same time. Relax. Repeat with your right arm and left leg. Relax. Repeat the entire exercise.

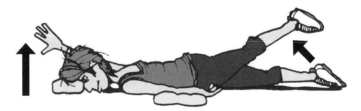

## 17. Elbow Prop

**Keep your head straight, eyes looking forward and your chin tucked in. A pillow under your stomach may help you feel more comfortable.**

Lie on your stomach. Keep both hands on the floor, by your face. With your elbows by your sides, slowly arch your back and pinch your shoulder blades together. While propped on your elbows, concentrate on relaxing the rest of your body. Hold for a count of 15, relax and repeat.

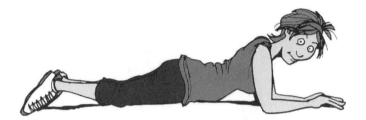

## 18. Kneel and Extend

**Do not arch up or down in your lower back. Also maintain your neck in a neutral position (keep your head and shoulders aligned, do not lower or raise your head).**

If you have been diagnosed with osteoporosis or you have any back or knee pain, do not do the following set of exercises without supervision of a physical therapist.

A. Start on your hands and knees. Place your knees and ankles together with your hands directly under your shoulders, your knees directly under your hips and your back straight.

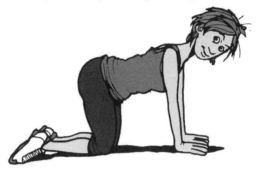

B. Lift your left arm to shoulder level and hold for three seconds. Return your hand to the floor directly under your left shoulder. Repeat with your right arm. Hold for three seconds. Your back should be straight, not sagging.

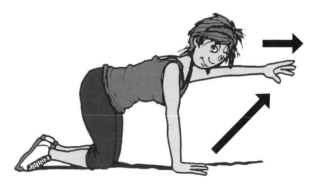

C. Slowly straighten your right leg and lift it to hip level. Hold for three seconds. Return your knee to the floor directly under your right hip. Repeat with your left leg. Do this only if you can do it comfortably without pain.

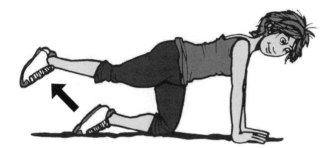

D. Slowly lift your left arm to shoulder level as you lift your right leg to hip level. Hold for three seconds. Relax. Repeat with your right arm and left leg.

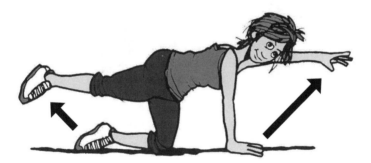

## 19. Corner Press Stretch

**Do not arch your back. This needs to be done very gently. You may feel a shoulder stretch. Avoid this exercise if it causes shoulder joint pain.**

Stand facing a corner, about eight inches or less away from the corner. Place one foot in front of the other and one hand on each wall at about ear level. With your back straight, bend forward from your ankles and very gently lean into the corner. Hold for a count of 15. Slowly push yourself back to an upright position. Relax and repeat.

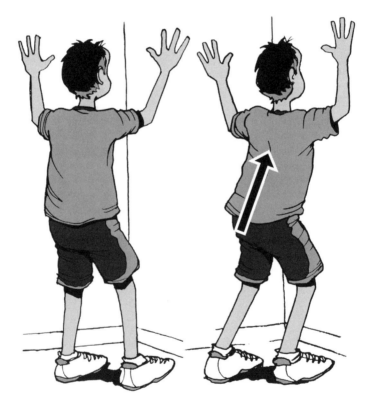

## 20. Shoulder Circles

Lift your left shoulder up while keeping your arm by your side. Slowly circle your left shoulder backward five times then return to the starting position. Repeat with the right shoulder.

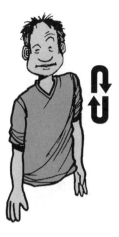

## 21. Side Stretch

**Do not twist your shoulders forward.**

Stand straight with feet firmly on the floor and arms at your sides. Pull your tummy in and slowly bend from your waist to the left side, with your left hand reaching as far down your left leg as possible. Slowly straighten your body and repeat on the right side. Repeat five times on each side.

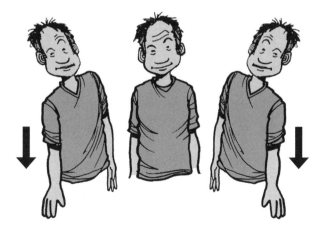

## 22. Shoulder Rotation

With your left elbow bent and tucked in at your side, slowly move your forearm away from your body as far as possible. Then bring your arm back in front of you and across your stomach. Relax and repeat with your right arm.

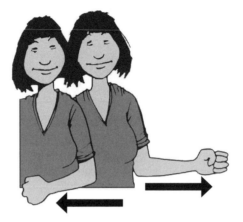

## 23. Shoulder Blade Pinch

**Do not push your head forward with your hands. If you have severe kyphosis, do this exercise gently and to the best of your ability. Avoid this exercise if it causes pain in your shoulders or back.**

With your chin pulled in, place your hands behind your ears and your elbows at or above shoulder level. Gently pinch your shoulder blades together. Hold for three seconds. Relax.

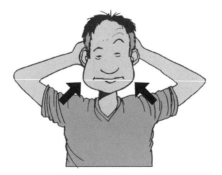

## 24. Hand Pull

Stand with your back against a wall. Bend your elbows and grip your hands firmly together at shoulder level. Bend your knees slightly and tighten your stomach muscles to flatten your spine against the wall. Gently try to pull your hands apart. Hold for a slow count of five. Relax.

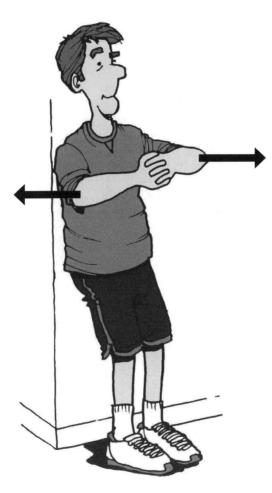

## 25. Arm Raises

With palms facing toward your legs, lift your arms out to the sides as high as your shoulders. Turn your palms up and lift your hands toward the ceiling. Slowly return your arms to the height of your shoulders. Turn your palms down and bring your arms back to your sides.

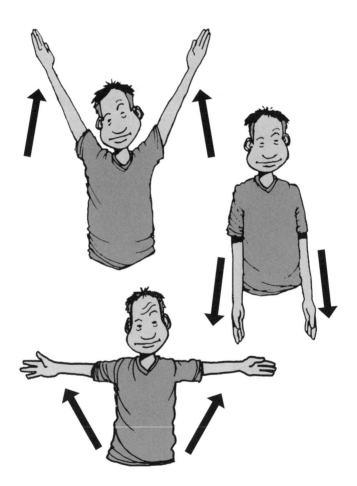

## 26. Wall Stretch

**Keep your chin tucked in and your tummy muscles tight to support and stabilize your lower back.**

Face the wall and stand with your toes about six inches from the wall. Take a deep breath as you stretch your right arm up the wall while stretching down with your left arm. Concentrate on gently stretching your upper back as you raise your arm and lean towards the wall. Hold for a count of five. Relax. Repeat with your left arm.

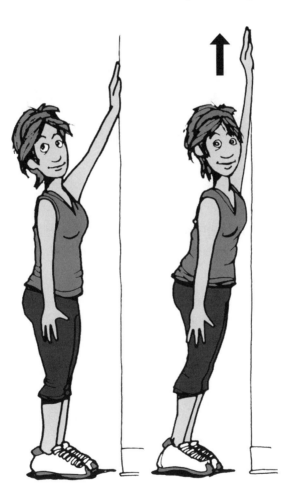

## 27. Neck

**Avoid bending your head backward or forward if you have rheumatoid arthritis or ankylosing spondylitis. If any dizziness occurs, return your head to the mid position and avoid this exercise.**

Look straight ahead with your chin tucked in. Drop your left ear to your left shoulder. DO NOT LET YOUR HEAD TWIST FORWARD. Slowly return your head to the center. Drop your right ear to your right shoulder and slowly lift your head to the center.

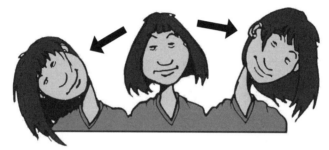

## 28. Head Turns

**Avoid bending your head backward or forward if you have rheumatoid arthritis or ankylosing spondylitis. If any dizziness occurs return your head to the mid position and avoid this exercise.**

Look straight ahead with your chin tucked in. Turn your head to the left so that you are looking over your left shoulder. No more than an 80 degree turn. Slowly turn to the right to look over your right shoulder. Turn back to the center.

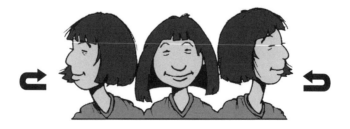

## 29. Toe Raise

**Keep your back straight, your seat tucked in and your tummy muscles tight.**

Stand facing a chair. Hold on to the back of the chair for support. Keeping your body straight, go up on your toes so that you lift your heels about six inches off the floor. Slowly return your heels to the floor. Rock back on to your heels and lift your toes off the floor. Slowly return your toes to the floor.

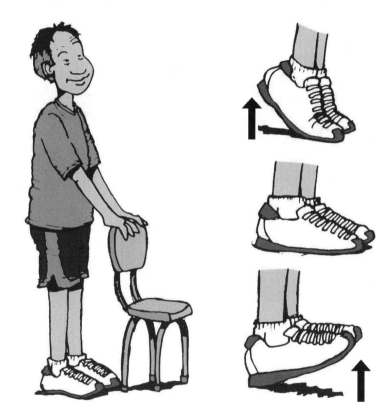

## 30. Rib Expansion and Relaxation

**Good for general relaxation**

Lie flat on your back. Relax with your shoulders down. Put your hands on your rib cage. Breathe in slowly for a count of three and feel your rib cage expand. Hold your breath for a moment. Then, as if to yawn, finish off with a final inhale "H" sound and exhale with a yawning sound "ahhhh." Be sure to push all the air out of your lungs and feel your rib cage collapse. Relax and repeat. Do this five times, then stop and rest for a minute. Repeat.

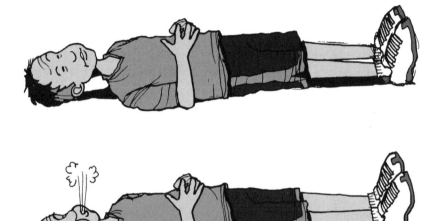

## 31. Tense and Relax

**Good for general relaxation. Breathe out while tightening your muscles.**

Lying flat on your back, breathe normally and systematically tighten all your muscles. First, curl your toes. Then tighten your knees, then your seat muscles and your shoulders. Close your eyes tight. Hold for a count of five and then relax your face, shoulders, seat, knees and finally your toes. Do not hold your breath.

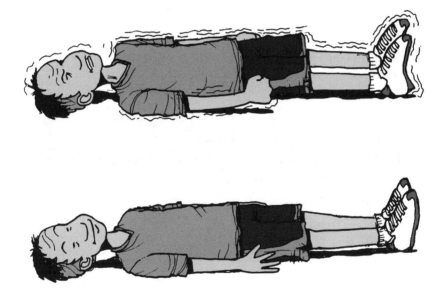

## SET B: BALANCE EXERCISES

Falling is a concern for older adults and even more so for anyone who has low bone density. If you are cautious and stiff when you move around, you are at a higher risk of falling than someone who moves easily and has good flexibility and balance. Ensuring optimal flexibility and balance is a very important part of the treatment for someone with osteoporosis.

Set B exercises are designed to improve balance. Be sure to exercise in a safe setting that is large enough so you do not bump into furniture, and the floor surface is safe and will not cause you to slip. Use a chair, sturdy table or countertop for support whenever it is appropriate.

It is important to move slowly and rhythmically when doing these exercises.

**Progress takes time, probably a few months.
Maintaining what you have until you improve is important,
so do not despair or give up.**

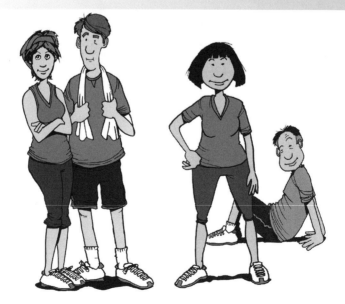

## 32. Heel and Toe Touches

Hold on to the back of a chair or counter for support. Stand with your hips pointing straight ahead. Touch the floor in front of you, first with your right heel and then with your left heel. Repeat 10 times, then touch the floor behind you, first with your right toe and then with your left toe.

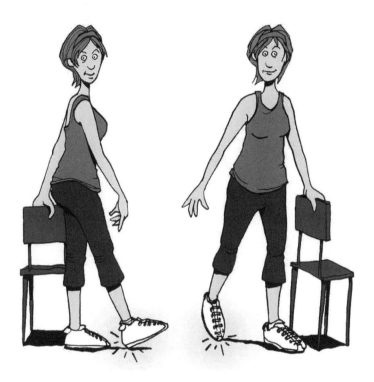

## 33. Sideways Leg Lift

**Keep your back straight, your seat tucked in and your tummy muscles tight.**

Stand behind a chair. Hold onto the back of the chair for support. With toes pointing forward, slowly lift your left leg sideways as far away from your body as you comfortably can. Repeat three times then repeat with your right leg. As you get better with this exercise, gradually ease your hold on the chair that you are using for balance. You may be able to do this exercise with only very light finger pressure on the chair back.

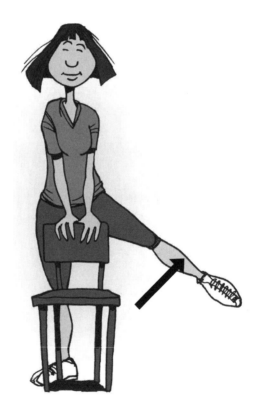

## 34. Side Step

**Keep your back straight, your seat tucked in and your tummy muscles tight.**

Stand straight, feet together. Move your right leg to the right about six inches. Bring your left leg over to the right leg. Now move your right leg over about six inches and bring your left leg over to the right leg. Repeat this three more times. Next, move your left leg to the left six inches and bring your right leg over to the left leg. Repeat this four times.

If you feel unsteady, rest your hands lightly on a support in front of you, such as a kitchen counter. As you improve with this exercise, try to put less and less pressure on the support.

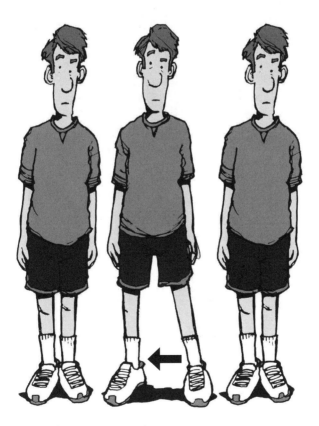

## 35. Arm Scissors

**Keep your back straight, your seat tucked in and your tummy muscles tight.**

Start with your arms low and by your sides. Use your arms like scissors. With your elbows straight, cross your left wrist over your right wrist and then reverse it by crossing your right wrist over your left wrist. As you do this, slowly raise your arms to chest level, then up to your ears. Continuing with the scissors motion, move your arms back to chest level and then to the low position. Slowly and gently repeat for up to one minute.

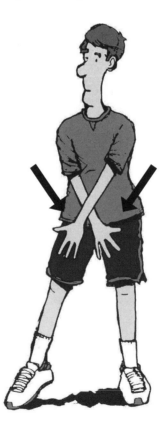

# 36. Marching

**Keep your back straight, your seat tucked in and your tummy muscles tight.**

A.  Stand in one spot and pretend to march slowly. Slowly raise your foot off the floor by bending one knee up in front of you as high as possible while keeping your stomach muscles tight and posture straight. Return your foot to the floor. Repeat with other foot and knee.

B.  Once you are comfortable doing the march, swing your left arm forward and back as you raise your right knee, then swing your right arm forward and back as you raise your left knee.

C.  As you march, raise both arms out to the side up to shoulder level if you can. Count to 10 and return your arms to your side. Slowly and gently repeat for up to one minute.

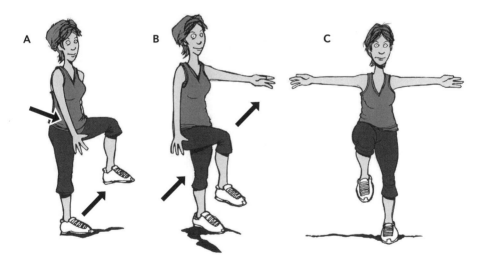

## 37. Gentle Sway

With your palms toward your legs, swing your arms forward and back. Stand with your feet apart and knees slightly bent. Transfer your weight from one foot to the other without lifting your feet off the ground, swaying from side to side. Repeat for one minute.

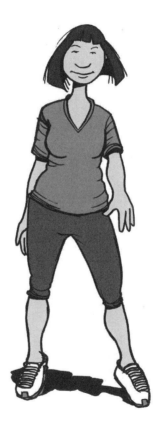

## 38. Air Punches

**Do this gently and rhythmically. Do not snap your elbow joints.**

Punch the air in front of you, first with your right hand then with your left. Next, punch towards your toes. Raise your arms to chest level and, with each arm, punch out to the side (away from your shoulder), then slowly back to the center. Slowly and gently repeat for up to one minute.

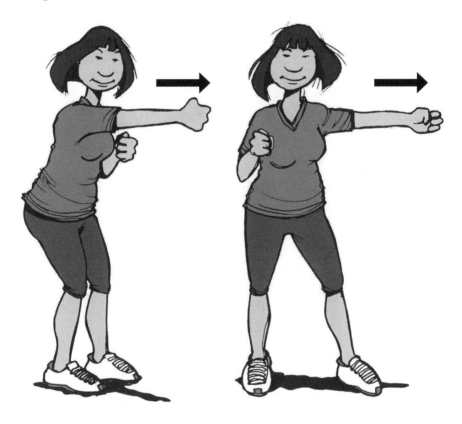

## 39. Elbow Bends as you Sway

Gently sway from side to side while you do this exercise. Start with your arms straight and by your sides. Bend your arms so that your fingers touch your shoulders and then straighten your arms again. Repeat three times and then start to move your arms up higher to the mid position (shoulder level). Reach to the shoulders and then straighten your arms. Finally, while still straightening and bending, lower your arms back down to your sides. Slowly and gently repeat for up to one minute.

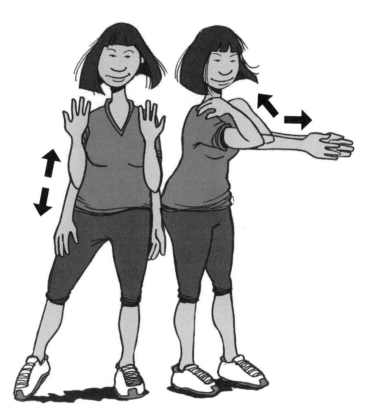

## 40. Arm Circles

Stand straight. Walk on the spot and raise both arms to shoulder level or to a level that is comfortable. Circle your arms forward. Draw small circles. Slowly make the circles smaller again. Now go in the other direction. Again, start with small circles and slowly make them bigger before working back to smaller circles.

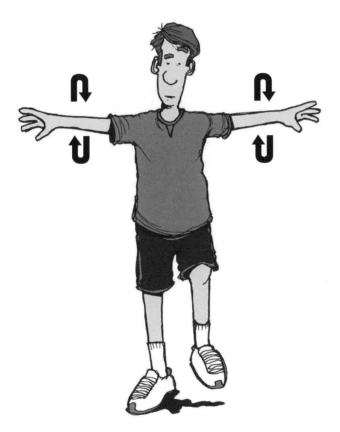

# CHAPTER 7 KEY POINTS

- Identify your risk of osteoporosis and fracture based on the assessment tests provided in the book. Complete the online FRAX test.

- Identify three exercises from each of the exercise sections, stretching, those that place stress on the spine and extremities, and balance.

- Develop a plan by completing the exercise chart with your doctor or physical therapist.

- Become familiar with the tips on how to move safely, especially when stretching, bending or lifting.

PART THREE

# Clinical Evaluations and Treatments

Clinical Evaluation to Assess Bone Health
10-Year Fracture Risk Assessment Tools
Fall and Fracture Prevention and Post Fracture Care
Medical Treatments
Understanding Health Headlines

# Clinical Evaluation to Assess Bone Health

Earlier in *The Osteoporosis Book* we learned that osteoporosis is characterized by impaired bone strength, which, in turn, increases a person's risk of broken bones (fractures). There are a number of reasons why people get osteoporosis, including:

- *Genetic inheritance*
- *Failure of bones to reach optimal peak bone mass*
- *Deterioration in the quality of bone*
- *Imbalance in the resorption and formation of bone that comes naturally with aging*
- *Other medical conditions or medications taken*
- *Combination of these causes*

If you have osteoporosis, you are at a higher risk of a fracture from a fall. Furthermore, it can have an adverse effect on your general state of health and well-being.

During your annual physical examination, a healthcare provider will generally take a medical history and do blood and urine tests. You will be checked for loss of height and changes in posture, the way you walk and your balance. Evaluations of bone health now include an assessment of both the risk for osteoporosis and the risk for fracture.

In Part 3 of *The Osteoporosis Book* we will look at what is involved in a typical clinical evaluation to assess bone health by reviewing your:

- *Risk factors for developing osteoporosis*
- *Risk of an osteoporosis-related fracture*
- *Need for a bone mineral density (BMD) test*

Using this information, you will be able to assess and evaluate your 10-year fracture risk. Later, we will review medical treatment options that will help you in making decisions on the best course of treatment for you. Together with your healthcare provider, review your findings and discuss your best options.

*If you or a loved one are over 50 and break a bone you should think osteoporosis. Follow-up by seeing your doctor for a comprehensive assessment and/or treatment for osteoporosis.*

## RISK FACTORS FOR OSTEOPOROSIS

## Review your risk of developing osteoporosis

We have listed risk factors for osteoporosis under three broad categories: family history, lifestyle, and medical history and medications. Check the factors that apply to you. Use this checklist with your healthcare provider to develop your care plan for the prevention and treatment of osteoporosis and related fractures.

### FAMILY HISTORY OR GENETICS

❑ *Age 50 or older*

❑ *Female*

❑ *Caucasian or Asian woman*

❑ *Low weight or body mass index less than 20kg/m2 (see glossary)*

❑ *Parent had hip fracture*

❑ *Loss of height 1.5 inches (4 cm) overall or 2.5 inches (6 cm) if over 60, when compared to the tallest height you were, or if you lost 1 inch (2.5 cm) in less than three years*

❑ *Low peak bone density*

## LIFESTYLE CHOICES

- ❑ Smoke tobacco products
- ❑ Drink excessive amount of alcohol (consistently three or more drinks per day)
- ❑ A woman who has excessive emotional or physical stress that disrupts or stops monthly periods
- ❑ Diet low in calcium or vitamin D
- ❑ Little exposure to sunlight, which may cause low vitamin D levels
- ❑ On extended bed rest or have an inactive lifestyle
- ❑ Caffeine is considered by some to be a small risk factor, particularly in the elderly who do not have enough calcium

## MEDICAL HISTORY AND MEDICATIONS

- ❑ History of glucocorticoid (prednisone) use
- ❑ Diagnosed with rheumatoid arthritis
- ❑ Diagnosed with celiac or other malabsorption disease
- ❑ Diagnosed with chronic liver or kidney disease
- ❑ Diabetes mellitus
- ❑ Medications include: antacids, anticoagulants, anti-depressants, anticonvulsants
- ❑ Estrogen/testosterone deficient
- ❑ Prostate or breast cancer medication
- ❑ Fractured a bone after age 45
- ❑ Kidney, thyroid, parathyroid, ovarian or liver problems
- ❑ Started menopause early (before age 45 years)
- ❑ Eating disorders, such as anorexia, bulimia

# RISK FACTORS FOR FALL AND FRACTURE

## Review your risk of a fall and an osteoporosis-related fracture

Various risk factors can contribute to osteoporosis-related fractures or broken bones. Bone loss is only one risk factor; your bone geometry or size and shape are also factors. Other factors include:

- ❏ *Age, the risk of fracture increases with age, especially at 65 years and older*

- ❏ *Decreased sight, hearing, balance or muscle strength*

- ❏ *Prior fragility (low trauma, low impact) fracture*

- ❏ *Poor health status – frail*

- ❏ *Balance – unstable on your feet*

- ❏ *Experienced a fracture after age 45*

- ❏ *Family history of osteoporotic fracture, for example: a direct relative had a hip fracture, higher risk if mother suffered a fracture*

- ❏ *Long-term use of glucocorticoid (more than three months continuously) therapy such as prednisone can affect your muscles and bones so they become weak*

- ❏ *Medications that affect your mobility and balance, such as sedatives*

- ❏ *Environmental hazards, such as uneven pavement on sidewalks, loose area rugs, poor lighting*

## WAYS TO ASSESS YOUR BONE HEALTH

## Bone Mineral Density Tests

- *Bone structure – generally only available in research studies by either taking a bone biopsy or using more advanced imaging technologies.*

- *Bone mineral density (BMD) – a measure of the amount of bone material in a defined area of bone, which will assist in the assessment of your fracture risk. The most common test used today is called dual energy X-ray absorptiometry (DXA).*

- *FRAX tool – developed by the World Health Organization to evaluate fracture risk.*

- *CAROC – Ten-Year Fracture Risk Assessment Tool. (FRAX and CAROC are discussed in more detail in Chapter 9.)*

- *Loss of height – greater than 1 inch (2.5 cm) within three years.*

- *Occiput-to-wall distance is greater than 2.5 inches (6 cm) and a rib to iliac crest distance of less than three finger widths, generally done by your doctor in his or her office.*

A BMD test measures the amount of bone in a defined area of bone. It does not show bone structure. Typically, if you had a BMD T-score (a number that indicates whether or not bone loss has occurred) below -2.5 SD (standard deviation), you would generally be treated for osteoporosis. However, many people with T-scores above -2.5 SD still fracture. Today, doctors are taking a broader view by focusing on ways to prevent fractures from occurring. To obtain a more complete bone assessment, doctors now use a BMD measurement along with an assessment of the osteoporosis and fracture risk factors referred to earlier to determine a person's osteoporosis status.

If you are at high risk of developing osteoporosis or show early signs of this condition (experienced height loss or a fracture for example), prevention and treatment measures should be considered. Discuss your medical history and current bone health with your doctor. Your risk assessment, together with a BMD measurement if necessary, will assist in assessing your current bone health and risk of future fracture.

BMD testing should be done to clarify risk of bone fracture and/or to assist in developing a care plan. Generally, older adults who take medications that cause thin or weakened bones are considered high risk and should be started on medications to prevent a fracture, without the need for a BMD test. Conversely, if the risk of fracture is sufficiently low, then a BMD test is not necessary. The predicted fracture risk will change as a person ages or develops new risk factors, at which time the need for a BMD test may be reconsidered (see the Bone Health Care Plan, p. 251).

The following list of indicators for BMD testing was developed by the International Society of Clinical Densitometry (ISCD). However, countries usually have their own guidelines defined by what specialists in those countries recommend and what is considered to be cost-effective by those involved in healthcare budgets and costs.

### ISCD INDICATORS FOR BMD TESTING

- *Women aged 65 and older*

- *Post-menopausal women under age 65 with risk factors for fracture*

- *Women during the menopausal transition with clinical risk factors for fracture, such as low body weight, prior fracture or high-risk medication use*

- *Men aged 70 and older (some experts say 65 years)*

- *Men under age 70 with clinical risk factors for fracture*

- *Adults with a low-trauma fragility fracture (fracture resulting from a fall from standing height or less)*

- *Adults with a disease or condition associated with low bone mass or bone loss (examples: anorexia, adrenal insufficiency, celiac disease, rheumatoid arthritis)*

- *Adults taking medications associated with low bone mass or bone loss (examples: corticosteroid such as prednisone, anticonvulsants such as phenytoin)*

- *Anyone prescribed pharmacologic therapy (drug therapy to prevent fractures) to monitor treatment effect*

- *Anyone not receiving therapy for whom evidence of bone loss would lead to treatment.*

Remember, there are many factors involved in measuring and interpreting a BMD test. BMD should be measured at a reliable clinic with a good quality control program. Ask if the technologists and physicians have had specific education in bone densitometry. Ideally, the machine being used should undergo quality assurance testing once a week and a service log should be maintained. The technologists should be tested periodically to ensure that the accuracy and reproducibility of their measurements are within acceptable limits.

It is your right to ask your technologist about the clinic's policy on maintaining the machines and the staff's continuing education. BMD measurements are susceptible to factors that can invalidate a measurement. An inaccurate BMD measurement is of no use.

How often a bone density should be repeated is an ongoing debate. If you are on high doses of glucocorticoid therapy or steroids, such as prednisone, testing may be done as often as every six months. You may also require bone density testing as a follow-up to determine if you are losing bone or if a treatment is working. The frequency of BMD tests should be determined using your risk factors and medical history.

Most experts feel that the average person with osteoporosis needs BMD testing usually no more than once every two years; sometimes three to five years is sufficient. After starting on medication to treat osteoporosis, it may take two or more years before significant changes in bone density occur. Measuring too soon may not allow sufficient time for changes to occur. Often, the absence of a fracture or absence of further decrease in bone density is good news and an indication that a medication is working. Don't be alarmed if your BMD result has not changed much since your last measurement. Remember that after about age 35, bone mineral density declines as you age. It is a positive sign if there is no change in your bone density. Talk with your healthcare provider about your personal situation.

If different machines are used to measure your bone density, you may see slightly different results. These differences do not affect diagnosis, but they may be important during follow-up when it becomes important to detect small changes. Therefore, if you have had a BMD test before, try to be retested on the same BMD machine whenever possible.

## BMD Accuracy

When a BMD test is conducted on a machine that is regularly calibrated and subject to quality assurance using proper techniques, the results should be accurate. Inaccuracies arise due to factors that may invalidate the measurement. For instance, if you wear clothing with zippers or clasps made of metal during a BMD test, the machine may interpret the metal as bone material. This could give a falsely elevated measurement. Osteophytes (bone spurs) and other calcifications on bone can also be falsely interpreted as bone mineral and result in a higher BMD measurement. A skilled densitometrist will recognize and account for these bone changes.

**The International Society of Clinical Densitometry (ISCD) has designations for qualified practitioners – Certified Clinical Densitometrist (CCD) or Certified Bone Densitometry Technologist (CBDT). An ISCD designation, achieved after passing an examination, is one way to determine if an individual involved with DXA testing or QUS testing has sufficient training and qualifications to perform these tests accurately.**

## Diagnostic Tools

The most common diagnostic tools used to determine an osteoporosis-related fracture are:

- *Plain radiography (X-ray)*

- *Computed tomography (CT) or magnetic resonance imaging (MRI)*

The most common diagnostic tools used to determine bone mineral density are:

- *Dual-energy X-ray absorptiometry (DXA)*
- *Quantitative computed tomography (QCT)*
- *Quantitative ultrasonography (QUS or ultrasound)*

### X-RAY

X-rays are usually used to diagnose back pain or spinal fracture. Before an X-ray will show bone loss, there must be at least a 40 percent loss of bone. Therefore, other methods are generally used to measure bone density. If you have a plain X-ray, ask the radiologist or your doctor to request that it be read for fracture as well as the original intent. Radiologists may not comment on fractures of the spine or bone density if not asked or if the X-ray was done for another reason. Because chest X-rays are common, they may provide valuable information about your spine that is not reported. Asking your doctor to add in the comment "rule out vertebral fracture" to any chest X-ray that is done for another reason will prompt the radiologist to note any visible fractures.

### CT or MRI

A CT or MRI may be used to clarify the findings on radiography rather than to provide bone density measurements. Your doctor may ask for this test if it is not clear from an X-ray whether or not you have a fracture.

### DXA

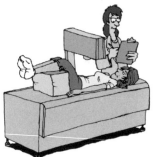

DXA is the most widely used test to measure bone density. DXA provides a very accurate measurement with very low radiation exposure. A DXA machine measures bone density by passing two very small beams of X-rays with differing energy levels through your bones. These beams measure the amount of bone

Dual-Energy X-ray
Absorptiometry (DXA)

material density. The different absorption levels of the two X-ray beams enable separate measurements to be taken of bone and soft-tissue density.

DXA is one of the easiest tests to take, as it does not involve swallowing anything or being given a needle. If you are not wearing any metal objects, such as a zipper, you do not even have to take off your clothes. The test usually measures bone density for your total hip, femoral neck, and lumbar spine (L1-L4). Bone density tests are read by a specialist who then provides a report to your healthcare provider.

A DXA test will provide a T-score. A T-score is a comparison of your bone density with that in young adults. These results are expressed as standard deviations (SD) and are derived from a standard reference database. Your T-score represents the number of standard deviations from the average normal peak bone mass around age 30.

This World Health Organization (WHO) classification of osteoporosis is based on T-scores of normal, low bone mass (osteopenia) or osteoporosis, was developed with DXA machines and a specific North American population. Based on this WHO classification, normal BMD is between -1 SD and +2 SD; low bone mass (osteopenia) is when the BMD is between -1 SD and –2.5 SD; and osteoporosis is when the BMD is -2.5 SD or less in post-menopausal women.

**A T-score of -1 SD means you have 10 to 15 per cent less bone than an average person at age 30. BMD decreases as we age, so -1 SD is considered normal and the risk of fracture is considered low.**

**A T-score of -1 SD to -2.4 SD means you have up to 25 per cent less bone than an average person at age 30 and you are at four times greater risk of fracture than the average young person.**

**A T-score of -2.5 SD or lower means you have at least 25 per cent less bone than an average person at age 30 and you are at eight times greater risk of fracture compared to that of an average young person.**

A T-score from other machines and other populations cannot be strictly compared. Although other technologies will produce a T-score, it does not equate with DXA T-scores and can be misleading.

Further research is required to understand fracture risk in men and pre-menopausal women. The criteria for diagnosing osteoporosis in these groups have not been well defined and doctors often use their clinical judgment in assessing the overall risk in these groups.

If you have had a previous fracture, your risk of fracturing again is two-fold or double compared with someone who has not had previous fracture. However, your other risk factors should be considered when determining your actual risk of fracture.

In some cases, usually for pre-menopausal women and for men, a BMD test will be reported as a Z-score. A Z-score cannot be compared to a T-score. A Z-score is matched to an average person your own age and is useful where enough data exist for comparison. A T-score is matched to an average person around the age of 30 and is generally thought to be the better method of reporting pre-menopausal women.

### QCT

Many QCT machines have software that measures the inner cancellous or spongy tissue of the bone in the vertebrae or spine, whereas the DXA machine looks at the whole bone. A QCT scan measures bone density, but unlike DXA, it does not use the standard database that provides the basis for the classification of a patient into the categories of normal or osteoporosis. QCT scans are expensive and results are based on a different database than DXA. Furthermore, QCT T-scores do not necessarily correspond to the WHO measurement standards (derived from DXA) to define normal and osteoporotic bone.

## QUS

Known as ultrasound, this technique is commonly available, but it has limitations. It is sometimes used as a secondary screening method, but it is not recommended for diagnosing osteoporosis.

- *For bone health, QUS is considered a screening method rather than a diagnostic method for osteoporosis (cannot reliably diagnose osteoporosis).*

- *QUS cannot be used to follow up the effects of treatment.*

- *When coupled with clinical risk factors, heel QUS can be used to identify individuals who are at seemingly low risk of fracturing, but it has limitations. Up to 10 percent of people who have a normal ultrasound should be aware that they may in fact have osteoporosis when their bone density is measured by a DXA bone mineral density test.*

- *QUS T-scores do not necessarily correspond to the WHO measurement standards (derived from DXA) to define normal and osteoporotic bone.*

Advantages of ultrasound are that it is relatively inexpensive and is portable so that it can be made available in various locations. There is no exposure to X-rays or radiation using ultrasound.

Ultrasound is more commonly used to measure bone density of the heel, wrist or part of the hand. Heel QUS, for example, often involves spreading a gel conductor on the ankle area and foot, then placing the foot in warm water and allowing the high frequency sound waves to pass through the heel. The intensity of the sound waves and their speed of transmission provide a measure of the bone density at that site. This technique is different from ultrasound that is used to diagnose gallstones, monitor pregnancy, etc.

# CHAPTER 8 KEY POINTS

- Family history or genetics, lifestyle choices, medical history and medications are all important when assessing your risk of osteoporosis.

- Aging, which can affect our sight, hearing, balance or muscle strength, medication use and history of previous fractures should be considered when evaluating our risk of falls and fractures.

- Bone density is not the same as bone quality.

- Bone mineral density (BMD) testing should be done to clarify fracture risk and/or to assist in developing a care plan (see the Bone Health Care Plan, p. 251).

- It is your right to ask your technologist about the clinic's policy on machine maintenance and the staff's continuing education. An inaccurate BMD is of no use.

- DXA (dual energy X-ray absorptiometry) is the most common test for measuring bone density.

- A T-score is a comparison of your bone density with that of a young adult. It was developed with a DXA machine in mind.

- A Z-score is matched to an average person your own age and is useful when enough data exists for a comparison.

- To accurately assess bone density, measure a baseline and then measure once every three years and compare the results. More frequent testing may be appropriate for some people.

- If you have a bone density test, try to be retested on the same machine.

- QUS (ultrasound) is used as a screening tool and not a tool for diagnosis, except in the less-developed world.

# 10-Year Fracture Risk Assessment Tools

## ASSESSING YOUR FRACTURE RISK

One of the biggest changes in the field of osteoporosis has been the use of FRAX and other fracture risk assessment tools to evaluate fracture risk of patients. These tools are a significant part of the clinical evaluation with your doctor or healthcare provider. They enable you to do your own risk assessment, which you can then review with your doctor or healthcare provider.

In this chapter, we will review two of these risk assessment tools: the web-based World Health Organization (WHO) Fracture Risk Assessment Tool commonly known as FRAX and the Canadian Association of Radiologists and Osteoporosis Canada (CAROC) system for fracture risk assessment.

Neither of these methods should be used for individuals under the age of 50. These methods are not accurate for estimating risk if a person has taken prescription osteoporosis treatments in the past or present.

## FRAX

FRAX uses a web-based questionnaire and calculation tool meant to be completed by a male or female between the ages of 40 and 90, either individually or with a healthcare provider, to assess a person's 10-year risk of osteoporosis fracture. Once the questions have been answered and your risk factors and other information are entered, the tool calculates your 10-year fracture probability as a percentage. The FRAX tool is designed for different countries and ethnic backgrounds.

FRAX is most effective when used by an operator who understands the significance of the questions being asked and can provide an accurate answer. A doctor may choose to use FRAX as an assessment tool prior to obtaining a bone density test or in conjunction with your results. If a BMD is not available, you can still use the FRAX tool by entering all other information including height and weight. By entering height and weight, your body mass index (BMI) can be calculated. If the FRAX risk is high, your healthcare provider may want to assess the level of bone loss with a bone mineral density test; if your risk is low, you may be advised to reuse the FRAX tool in one year, provided nothing changes during that time.

## FRAX Questionnaire*

### RISK FACTORS IN THE FRAX CALCULATOR

For most risk factors, choose a yes or no response. If the field is left blank, then a "no" is assumed. It is important to note this calculator is only applicable for those who have not taken prescription therapies for osteoporosis in the past or present.

1. *Age: the model accepts ages between 40 and 90 years. If ages below or above are entered, the program will compute probabilities at 40 and 90 years, respectively.*

2. *Sex: Male or female. Enter as appropriate.*

3. *Weight: This should be in kilograms (1 kg = 2.2 lb). To convert pounds to kg, divide the number of pounds by 2.2 or use the conversion calculator provided with the online calculation tool.*

4. *Height: this should be entered in centimeters (2.54 cm = 1 inch). To convert inches to cm, multiply number of inches by 2.54 or use the conversion calculator provided with the online calculation tool.*

*\* Adapted with permission of the WHO Collaborating Centre for Metabolic Bone Diseases, University of Sheffield. FRAX® is registered to Professor J.A. Kanis, University of Sheffield. (GE Lunar, Hologic, or Norland DXA scanners). The FRAX questionnaire is reproduced here for information only. To properly use FRAX to calculate your 10-year risk of osteoporosis fracture, refer to the online calculator tool available at www.sheffield.ac.uk/FRAX/*

5. *Previous fracture: A previous fracture denotes more accurately a previous fracture in adult life occurring spontaneously, or fracture arising from trauma which, in a healthy individual, would not have resulted in a fracture. Enter yes or no. (see also notes below on risk factors)*

6. *Parent fractured hip: this enquires for a hip fracture in the patient's mother or father. Enter yes or no*

7. *Current smoking: enter yes or no depending on whether the patient currently smokes tobacco. (see also notes below on risk factors)*

8. *Glucocorticoids: Enter yes if the patient is exposed to oral glucocorticoids or has been exposed to oral glucocorticoids for more than 3 months at a dose of prednisolone (prednisone) of 5mg daily or more (or equivalent doses of other glucocorticoids)(see also notes below on risk factors)*

9. *Rheumatoid arthritis: enter yes where the patient has a confirmed diagnosis of rheumatoid arthritis. Otherwise enter no.*

## Calculation Tool

Please answer the questions below to calculate the ten year probability of fracture with BMD.

Country: Canada          Name/ID: [          ]          About the risk factors (i)

### Questionnaire:

1. Age (between 40-90 years) or Date of birth

| Age: | Date of birth: |
| 60 | Y: 1950  M: 06  D: 06 |

2. Sex                   ○ Male  ◉ Female

3. Weight (kg)           [ 62 ]

4. Height (cm)           [ 140 ]

5. Previous fracture     ○ No  ◉ Yes

6. Parent fractured hip  ◉ No  ○ Yes

7. Current smoking       ◉ No  ○ Yes

8. Glucocorticoids       ○ No  ◉ Yes

9. Rheumatoid arthritis  ◉ No  ○ Yes

10. Secondary osteoporosis    ◉ No  ○ Yes

11. Alcohol 3 or more units per day  ◉ No  ○ Yes

12. Femoral neck BMD (g/cm²)

[ T-Score ▼ ]  [ -2 ]

[ Clear ]          [ Calculate ]

BMI: 31.6
The ten year probability of fracture (%)

with BMD

| ■ Major osteoporotic | 21 |
| ■ Hip fracture | 3.3 |

**Frax Calculation Tool**

10. Secondary osteoporosis: enter yes if the patient has a disorder strongly associated with osteoporosis. These include type 1 (insulin dependent) diabetes, osteogenesis imperfecta in adults, untreated long-standing hyperthyroidism, hypogonadism or premature menopause (before age 45), chronic malnutrition, or malabsorption and chronic liver disease.

11. Alcohol 3 or more units/day: Enter yes if the patient takes 3 or more units of alcohol daily. A unit of alcohol varies slightly in different countries from 8 to 10g of alcohol. This is equivalent to a standard glass of beer (285ml), a single measure of spirits (30ml), a medium-sized glass of wine (120ml), or 1 measure of an aperitif (60ml).

12. Bone mineral density (BMD): Select the maker of the DXA scanning equipment used and enter the actual femoral neck BMD (in g/cm2). For patients without a BMD test, the field should be left blank. The drop-down box enables you to enter a T-score as an option.

## Notes on Risk Factors

### PREVIOUS FRACTURE
A special situation pertains to a prior history of vertebral fracture. A fracture detected as a radiographic observation alone (a morphometric vertebral fracture) counts as a previous fracture. A prior clinical vertebral fracture from which the patient suffers consequences, such as pain, is an especially strong risk factor. The probability of fracture computed may, therefore, be underestimated. Fracture probability is also underestimated in the yes/no scenario as the risk of multiple fractures is greater than single fractures.

### SMOKING, ALCOHOL, GLUCOCORTICOIDS
These risk factors appear to have a dose-dependent effect (i.e., the higher the exposure, the greater the risk). This is not taken into account and the computations assume average exposure. Clinical judgment should be used for low or high exposures.

### RHEUMATOID ARTHRITIS (RA)

RA is a risk factor for fracture. However, osteoarthritis is, if anything, protective. For this reason, reliance should not be placed on a patient's report of arthritis unless there is clinical or laboratory evidence to support the diagnosis.

### BONE MINERAL DENSITY (BMD)

The site and reference technology is DXA at the femoral neck. T-scores are based on the NHANES reference values for women aged 20-29 years. The same absolute values are used in men as gender is accounted for in the FRAX calculation tool.

50% of hip fracture patients will suffer another fracture within five years. Be sure to follow-up with a comprehensive assessment and/or treatment for osteoporosis after any fracture.

If your mother or father broke a hip, you are at a higher risk of osteoporosis.

## CAROC FRACTURE RISK ASSESSMENT

The CAROC Fracture Risk Assessment system (Figure 1) was developed by the Canadian Association of Radiologists and Osteoporosis Canada. Fracture risk assessment is based upon gender, age, BMD at the femoral neck, prior fragility fracture, and glucocorticoid use. Fracture risk is categorized as low (less than 10 percent), moderate (10-20 percent) or high (more than 20 percent). To use this method to determine your 10-year fracture risk:

1. *Select the appropriate table – women or men.*

2. *Select the column that is closest to your age*

3. *Determine your fracture risk category by using the femoral neck T-score from your BMD measurement.*

4. *Determine your fracture risk by looking at age, gender, fracture history and glucocorticoid use. Intersect your age and femoral neck T-score. Move up one risk level if you have had a fragility fracture or are on long-term steroid use.*

Based on results of low, moderate or high risk of fracture, your doctor can identify your best course of treatment. A repeat risk assessment is appropriate in 10 years for people with low risk and in one to five years for people with moderate or high risk

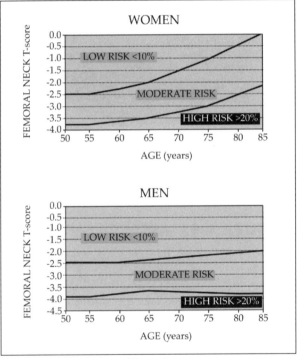

**Figure 1**

**Figure 1:** *Assessment of basal 10-year risk of fracture with the 2010 tool of the Canadian Association of Radiologists and Osteoporosis Canada. The T-score for the femoral neck should be derived from the National Health and Nutrition Education Survey III reference database for white women. Fragility fracture after age 40 or recent prolonged use of systemic glucocorticoids increases the basal risk by one category (i.e., from low to moderate or moderate to high). This model reflects the theoretical risk for a hypothetical patient who is treatment naive; it cannot be used to determine risk reduction associated with therapy. Individuals with a fragility fracture of a vertebra or hip and those with more than one fragility fracture are at high risk of an additional fracture. (Adapted with permission from CAROC)* (risk assessment by your doctor will be needed if treated with prescription osteoporosis treatment). As with the FRAX calculator tool, the CAROC method of estimating the 10-year risk of fracture is only applicable to people who have not received any prescription osteoporosis therapies. Both of these methods can be used if you are taking or have taken vitamin D and/or calcium supplements.

Try doing your own risk fracture assessment. Use the FRAX tool, which you can find on the website of the World Health Organization (or search the internet for FRAX) or follow the CAROC fracture risk assessment tool in this chapter. Once you have determined your risk over 10 years, you can decide whether or not you want to take medication. Experts suggest that if you are at low risk, then you do not need medication and should treat with appropriate lifestyle changes. If your risk is moderate, you might consider treatment in addition to lifestyle changes. However, if your 10-year fracture risk is high, you probably would benefit from a medication and you should consider making lifestyle changes. Review your assessment with your doctor to establish your bone health status and best treatment options given your full medication history (see the Bone Health Care Plan, p. 251).

## CHAPTER 9 KEY POINTS

- **If you break a bone through normal movements or a low-energy fall, you likely have osteoporosis and should have a risk assessment for future fractures done by your doctor.**

- **Your 10-year fracture risk can be estimated by using the online-based FRAX tool or CAROC tool.**

- **Fracture risk assessment can help you to identify your best treatment plan.**

# CHAPTER 10

# Fall and Fracture Prevention and Post-Fracture Care

**When an adult fractures a bone – think osteoporosis!**

A significant part of a clinical evaluation is the assessment of your risk of a fall. Falls are the most common cause of injury among the elderly. They account for 40 percent of elderly admissions into nursing homes and long-term care facilities. A fall can result in fear of falling again. This fear may result in restricted or cautious movements and doing activities that, in turn, can increase the risk of falling again. This chapter looks at factors that may affect your risk of falling. We also will look at the gap in care when all too often the doctors and patients fail to connect a fracture with osteoporosis.

## FALL PREVENTION

More than one-third of adults over the age of 65 fall each year. One-third of people who fall suffer moderate to severe injuries such as bruising, head trauma or hip fractures. These injuries can lead to a reduced quality of life through limited movement, a stay in a nursing home or premature death. Studies have shown that osteoporosis is a factor in up to 80 percent of hip fractures.

The first objective in preventing fractures is to prevent a fall from occurring. To this end, safeguard your environment and do your exercises targeted at improving balance.

The second objective is to prevent a fracture from occurring if you fall. By having the best bone density, structure and quality of bone, you will reduce your risk of fracture from a fall.

# Factors that Increase Your Risk of Falling

## AGING

As we age, physical changes occur in our bodies. Around age 60 we experience:

- **Eyesight changes.** *We cannot see as well in low light and we lose some depth perception. As a result, we may not be able to see a potential problem, such as an obstacle in our way or a step in front of us.*
  *Tip: Have regular eye check-ups. If you have prescription glasses, be sure to wear them. Carry a small pocket-sized high-powered flashlight to help you see obstacles in your path.*

- **Inner ear changes.** *Changes in our ears can result in a slight decrease in our balance and increase how much we sway. A decrease in hearing can change awareness of your environment.*
  *Tip: Have regular hearing check-ups.*

- **Muscle changes.** *As we age, muscles lose flexibility and strength. If our muscles are weak, they may not be able to support our body's frame. If you are stiff and inflexible, your body may not be able to adjust to unexpected situations, such as uneven ground or others' quick movements.*
  *Tip: Follow a regular exercise program that you have discussed with your doctor.*

- **Response time changes.** *Our reflexes slow down so that we cannot recover as quickly if we stumble.*
  *Tip: Be aware of your movements and stay focused.*

## DISEASES

- **Joint problems**, *such as arthritis of the toes, feet, ankles, knees or hips, may cause you to walk incorrectly. You may walk with a shuffle, take shorter steps or swing your arms less, all of which may affect your balance.*
  *Tip: Pick up your feet when you walk. Be sure to do your balance exercises.*

- **Cardiovascular (heart) problems** can increase the occurrence of postural hypotension (a lowering of pressure when moving from a lying or sitting position to standing too quickly, so that you become lightheaded or dizzy).
  **Tip:** Move slowly when changing positions, do not rush. When sitting up from a lying position, pause for a moment before standing.

- **Central nervous system problems**, such as multiple sclerosis or Parkinson's disease, may cause poor balance. A person with dementia may forget where a chair is and miss it as they sit down.
  **Tip:** Use mobility aids as necessary.

- **Diabetes** may decrease the sharpness or acuity of your senses so that you are not as aware of your surroundings. Most commonly affected are the eyes and feet.
  **Tip:** Manage diabetes as directed to decrease the negative effects.

- **Nerve damage.** If you have nerve damage in your feet, your feet will not be as sensitive to position and balance.
  **Tip:** Wear properly fitted shoes, ensure proper foot care as directed and use mobility aids as necessary.

- **Eye disease** may impair your assessment of depth and distance of sidewalk changes and curbs.
  **Tip:** Mobility aids may help you be aware of your surroundings and help steady you as you move. A pocket flashlight may help to increase your visibility as you walk.

## MEDICATIONS

- **Effects of certain medications**, such as antidepressants and blood pressure medications, can make you lightheaded, dizzy or tired and cause you to lose your balance. Sleeping pills may make you drowsy, which can increase your risk of falling when you wake up to go to the bathroom or kitchen at night.
  **Tip:** Medications should be taken as directed and with caution. Check with your doctor and pharmacist to find out about any side effects or interactions. If a sleeping pill makes you feel too groggy or slow in the morning, check with your doctor and

*pharmacist about a shorter-acting, more appropriate medication. Be sure to follow instructions when taking any medication ("take only at bedtime" or "do not operate machinery, a car, etc.").*

- **Review your medication** *with your family doctor or healthcare provider on a regular basis.*
  **Tip:** *Medications should be reviewed at your annual physical and assessed for their need or value. Discuss the medications prescribed by your specialists to see that they are still effective and necessary. Tell your pharmacist about all the medications – prescription and over-the-counter, including herbal remedies – as they could interact.*

## ENVIRONMENTAL FACTORS

- **Floors and stairs.** *It is easy to trip on a loose rug or catch the toe of your shoe on a stair.*
  **Tips:** *Maintain surfaces, both indoors and outdoors, in good repair (no loose boards or carpet). Install hand rails on stairs. Securely fasten all rugs on floors and stairs. Remove threads or tassels from rugs.*

- **Bedrooms and Bathrooms.** *Many falls happen on the way to or in the bathroom. We know the bathroom is just around the corner and we know the way, but the bathroom is often slippery and dark.*
  **Tips:** *Keep bed coverings up off the bedroom floor and shoes put away. Turn a light on so you can see your way to the bathroom. Install grab bars to steady yourself when stepping in and out of the tub. Apply non-skid tape or decals in the bathtub or use a rubber bath mat. Use a rubber-backed bath mat to prevent slipping on a wet floor when you are getting out of the tub.*

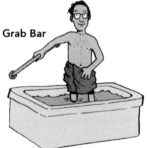

Grab Bar

- **Lighting.** *Poorly lit or unfamiliar areas where you cannot see the floor or your surroundings, such as outdoor areas, restaurants or even your home in the middle of the night, are dangerous.*

*Tips:* Use bright lights indoors and outdoors. Ensure that light switches on lamps are easy to reach. When up during the night, put on your glasses and turn on the light so you can see where you step. Install small sensor lights that turn on automatically when you walk through hallways and bathrooms. Use a flashlight to help you see your way. Use a bathroom night light or a low wattage bathroom light.

- *Around the house.* Pets, small children, power cords or other items left on the floor are easy to trip over.
  *Tips:* Be sure there are no cords from lamps, televisions, heaters, etc., to trip over. Clean up spills immediately. Be cautious with pets around your feet. Be sure your shoes are secure, avoid backless slippers and find shoes that will stay on your whole foot.

- *Outdoors.* Uneven pavement, cracks in pavement or varying curb heights are potential problems. Wet surfaces or walking on snow, ice or leaves can result in a slip.
  *Tips:* Be cautious when walking on snow, ice or leaves. You may even try crampons or ice grips, which are spikes that go over your shoes (be sure to take them off when you go indoors – they can be slippery on indoor surfaces). Watch where you walk and, if possible, walk on even ground. Use solid, sturdy shoes with low, broad heels for stability

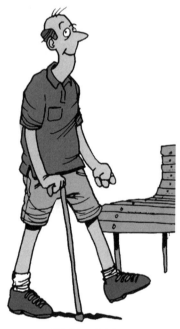

**Walking Stick**

when walking. An oxford style shoe with a rubber sole and heel or running shoes with proper support are invaluable. If you must

*wear a dress shoe, be sure it has a low, broad heel. Check for heel*
*support so that there is no tendency to twist over on your ankle.*
*Use mobility aids, such as walking sticks, canes and walkers as*
*necessary. Be social and walk holding onto a friend.*

Changes in our physical condition can be slow and subtle as we
age. Be sure you know your own risk factors. Use the "Get Up and
Go Test" in the glossary or consult with your healthcare provider
to do a fall risk assessment, especially if you have previously
suffered a fall. Identify, address and correct your risk factors for
falls as much as possible.

## FRACTURE PREVENTION

**Statistics reinforce the need for us to be informed consumers and
our own best advocates. Ask questions, find out what is needed
and follow up to ensure that it has happened.**

Keeping muscles strong and staying agile and supple will help
to prevent falls and fractures from occurring. Because an older
person has lower bone density, resulting in weaker bones, the
amount of stress required to cause a fracture may be much less
than for a younger person. A small fall or even an unexpected
twist can result in a fracture, which is why balance and balance
exercises are very important as we age.

If you fall, your risk of fracture may depend on one or more of
the following:

- *Your height*

- *The distance of your fall*

- *Any protective response, such as putting your hand out to
  break a fall*

- *The type of surface on which you fall*

- *The angle in which you fall; falling sideways or straight down is more risky than falling backwards*

- *Bone geometry or shape and density of your bone*

- *Whether or not you were wearing a good hip protector that fits properly*

## Wrist

Wrist fractures are more common at an earlier age and stage of osteoporosis. They often happen when the arm is extended to break a fall. Although not usually disabling, such fractures can serve as a warning that excessive bone loss may be occurring or there may be a more serious fracture in the future. Take this opportunity to further investigate your bone health. Do not let a wrist fracture occur without following up to determine if you have osteoporosis and what your risk is of another fracture.

## Spine

Bone loss in the spine may cause the vertebrae to become weak and porous. If bone loss continues, vertebrae may become so thin that they eventually collapse (fracture) under the weight of the body, perhaps during a simple, everyday movement like turning to look behind you.

Vertebral fractures can result in height loss and can cause serious concerns with respect to body organs (such as those involved with breathing or digestion), changes in body image, independence, self-esteem and quality of life. After you have had an osteoporotic vertebral fracture, your risk of having a hip fracture doubles. Early detection and treatment is key to preventing future fractures. Amazingly, 65 percent of people who have these types of fractures do not experience symptoms such as pain.

## Keep Track of Your Height

Since height loss may be an indicator of osteoporosis and fractures in the spine, you can easily measure your own height between doctor's visits. Talk with your doctor about a spinal fracture if you have a height loss of:

- *1.5 inches (4 cm) since your tallest known height and are under the age of 60*
- *2.5 inches (6 cm) since your tallest known height and you are over the age of 60*
- *greater than 1 inch (2.5 cm) in the last three years*

Although height loss is a simple and valuable way to detect vertebral fractures, it does not pick up all the fractures or specify the type of fracture, such as a wedge or collapse.

## Chest X-ray

The good news is that spinal fractures or collapse can be identified on a chest X-ray or other radiograph. A patient can request that the bone health of the spine be checked when an X-ray is ordered. Some experts suggest that every chest X-ray should be read for bone health of the spine even if the chest X-ray was ordered for another reason. If a spinal fracture or collapse is evident, it should then be treated to prevent future fractures.

One study of women over age 60 who had a spine X-ray for a reason other than suspected fracture (for example, a chest X-ray for pneumonia) found that although almost half the women had spinal fractures, only 19 percent were identified and treated. When having a chest X-ray for any reason, ask your doctor to request "rule out vertebral fracture."

The bad news is that spinal fractures are an important indicator of osteoporosis and risk of future fractures, yet they may be missed. Some larger hospitals, teaching facilities and major osteoporosis clinics have bone density machines that produce images of the spine at the time of measuring bone mineral density. These images, along with monitoring a patient's height, help promote early detection of spinal fractures and lead to treatment that decreases the risk of future fractures.

If treatment for the prevention of future fractures is not started, a cascade of spinal fractures or even a hip fracture is likely to follow.

Patients can have four to five fractured or collapsed vertebrae without pain and show a hump (kyphosis) before an obvious sign is seen and their spine is investigated. It is important to keep a check on the curve of your spine and your height from year to year.

## Hip Fractures

Hips fractures are associated with significant morbidity (where the person develops a sickness or disease) and mortality (where the person dies). The death rate within five years of a hip fracture is about 20 percent higher than the death rate for people without a fracture. Remember, this group is elderly, so their longevity is shorter, but quality of life is always important.

Of the individuals who return to their communities following a hip repair, only 30 percent receive osteoporosis evaluation and treatment. The 70 percent that are not evaluated for osteoporosis have a significant chance of fracturing the other hip. If you have had a hip or other fracture and are not currently on treatment, discuss with your doctor how to prevent further fractures.

## Mobility Aids

If you are unsteady on your feet and have a fear of falling, you have some choices. You can remain active by using a mobility aid to provide safer, more secure movement, or you can accept a less physically active life with fewer social interactions and a reduced quality of life. Tough choices yes.

For some, the thought of using a cane, for example, creates images of being old, frail or disabled. It can make even the strongest person feel inadequate and frustrated. It can remind us that we are not the person we once were. So we can choose to sit still, pretend we are okay and deny our situation.

Mobility aids, on the other hand, support our abilities should we choose to maintain our independence and quality of life. Using a mobility aid gives us more freedom to be active and independent. It implies that we want to be safe – things we should celebrate.

Aids such as sturdy shoes, walking sticks, canes, walkers, scooters and electric or hand powered wheelchairs provide safer movement if used properly. These aids come in a variety of styles, so choose one that fits your personality or the occasion. Many specialty shoe stores have experts trained in fitting people with mobility issues. Walking sticks are now used by people of all ages to provide a little extra stability over uneven ground. Canes come in different handles, lengths and colors. They may be wood or metal, hand-carved or graphic; some are equipped with special grips for snow and ice. Norwegian hiking poles can project an image of fitness while providing stability. Some people carry poles or canes to protect themselves from crowds or pets. For others, they make a fashion statement. Many walkers come with an optional seat so you can sit when a line-up is too long or moves too slowly. Some walkers have carry baskets for when you are shopping. They can be lightweight, easy to maneuver and easily stored. If you live in a home with stairs and do not want to move, consider the cost of a stair lift. It can be a lot less expensive than a move. Imagine the freedom these aids provide.

There are right and wrong ways for using any device. Be sure you get the proper instructions for using any mobility device. Be careful not to trip over the device as you get used to taking it with you. Most important, use it. As statistics show, a fall can be a life altering event that may result in a fracture, loss of independence and sometimes death. At the very least, a mobility aid can improve your confidence when walking.

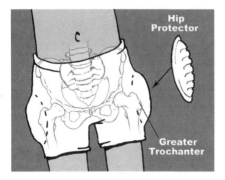

## Hip Protectors

A hip protector is a device worn as an undergarment that offers additional protection against a hip fracture. The undergarment has a pad, either hard or soft, that rests over the hip area, specifically the greater trochanter. Be sure it is positioned properly. If you fall, the hip protector is designed to absorb and disperse the energy from the impact of the fall away from the hip bone to the soft tissue and muscle around the hip bone.

Although clinical research is inconclusive, some studies suggest that hip protectors can reduce the risk of a fractured hip from falling by 50 percent. Hip protectors are constantly improving and are available in many styles. If you have not looked at hip protectors recently, be sure to check them out. Hip protectors only work if you wear them properly!

A note of caution, it has been reported that individuals have occasionally fallen while taking off hip protectors, so be careful.

## POST-FRACTURE CARE

**A fracture means you are at high risk of osteoporosis and a second fracture. All fractures for people over age 45 should be investigated for osteoporosis.**

Research has shown less than 20 percent of women and 10 percent of men are appropriately tested and treated after a fragility or osteoporotic fracture. After a broken bone has been repaired and before you leave the hospital, there are some things you might request to help your recovery and enable you to return to your quality of life.

Ideally, after a broken bone from a low-trauma fracture, you would be treated in hospital and given a case manager. Your case manager will work with you to develop a treatment and follow-up plan. The surgical report should have been sent from your orthopedic surgeon to your doctor (see the Bone Health Care Plan, p. 251). It is important to have a doctor or healthcare provider that can oversee your care path and recovery. If you are diagnosed with osteoporosis, discuss coping strategies and resources for managing a chronic illness, such as educational resources, family, friends and local support groups.

The care plan may include a healthcare team comprising a physical therapist, dietitian, home care nurse, pharmacist, family doctor and osteoporosis specialist. If this does not happen, put your own plan in place. Use a binder or multi-pocket file to hold information as you receive it.

Your care plan might include:

- *Post-operation Wound Care – wound care, bandage changes and stitches or staple removal 10 to 14 days after surgery at the doctor's office, a clinic or at home by a home care worker.*

- *Rehabilitation, including a physical therapist, education about maintaining bone health, mobility aids, fall risks, keeping a safe environment, available support in the community, development of an appropriate, manageable, long-term exercise program.*

- *Pain medications – see Chapter 14 regarding pain management.*

- *Medication review: to assess your general health status and ensure medications and other disease issues are not contributing to your bone loss or the risk of falling; to discuss how to reduce your risk of a future fracture; and, if appropriate, to identify your treatment for osteoporosis.*

- *Diet review to assess and supplement, if necessary, your daily dietary intake of calcium, vitamin D and other valuable nutrients.*

- *Further testing, such as blood work, vitamin D level testing, tests to rule out secondary causes of osteoporosis, BMD test.*

- *Referral to a specialist in osteoporosis.*

- *Review and address any factors related to aging, disease, medication and environment that increase your risk of falling.*

As part of your post-fracture care plan, be sure to follow-up with your doctor. If you have a healthcare team in place, work with the team members to maintain and improve your bone health.

Studies have shown there are gaps in care for bone health. We know that as few as 20 percent of people receive the treatment they need. With a little education and awareness, you can prevent many first and second fractures or at least decrease your risk of fracture and their impact on the quality of life of you and your family. Be sure to contact your national, state, provincial or local bone health organizations or an osteoporosis clinic for help in finding the best possible follow-up care.

## CHAPTER 10 KEY POINTS

- **If you break a bone after age 45, think osteoporosis and follow up with your doctor.**
- **Less than 20 percent of women and 10 percent of men are appropriately tested after an osteoporotic-related fracture.**
- **Be aware of the effects that age, disease, medications, lifestyle and environment may have on your risk of falling.**
- **Keeping your muscles strong, agile and supple will help prevent falls and fractures.**
- **Be aware of your height and any height loss as loss may signal osteoporosis of the spine.**
- **If you have a regular spinal or chest X-ray, ask your doctor to "rule out vertebral fracture."**
- **Take steps to prevent another fall and fracture. Exercise and use osteoporosis medication and mobility aids such as canes or walkers as necessary.**
- **If you fracture, set up a care plan to help ensure a full recovery.**

# CHAPTER 11
# Medical Treatments

The goal of drug therapy is to reduce fracture risk by preventing further bone loss and promoting strong bones. People with severe osteoporosis are more likely to make the decision to take a drug after a significant fracture has occurred. But for someone who is at an earlier stage of the disease with mild to moderate bone loss or who is considering ways to prevent osteoporosis, the decision about whether or not to take a drug may be more difficult.

Choosing the right drug can be a challenge as different medications provide different benefits and, in some cases, side effects. Some drugs assist in preventing bone loss while others are approved for treatment of low, moderate and severe bone loss. Some medications have a greater impact on the spine while others also impact the hip.

Drugs that have been approved by national health authorities for general use in disease-specific situations are considered established therapies. In the United States, the Food and Drug Administration (FDA) assesses the results of studies and decides whether or not to approve drug therapies that have been found to be safe and effective. In Canada, this is done by the Therapeutic Products Directorate (TPD).

This chapter will help you to understand the range of drug therapies available for preventing or managing osteoporosis, and, most importantly, for preventing fractures. It will identify how drugs work – in other words their mechanisms of action (MOA). We will discuss how drugs get into your body, known as the route of administration. You will be encouraged to weigh the benefits, risks and costs associated with taking medications in relation to your own health situation. Finally, we will describe possible side effects and rare events of taking specific drugs.

## MECHANISM OF ACTION

When considering a drug's mechanism of action (MOA), or how the drug works, we look at the way a drug produces an effect on the body. Drugs can have different mechanisms of action through which they can help to improve bone density. Improved bone density assists in reducing fracture risk.

Drugs fall under four general categories:

- *Anti-resorptive drugs slow down bone removal by inhibiting the osteoclast cells. "Anti" means against and "resorptive" means to suck in or remove by resorption. By slowing down the action that removes bone material, bone thinning is slowed.*

- *Anabolic (building) drugs assist in bone formation by stimulating the osteoblast cells. These drugs act on osteoblast cells to speed up bone formation.*

- *RANKL inhibition can be accomplished by using a human antibody that binds to RANKL and inhibits the RANKL pathway. It has an anti-resorptive mechanism of action with the added benefit of having a more direct way to slow bone breakdown. The drug will interfere with the function of a protein. This protein is known as Receptor Activator for Nuclear Factor κB Ligand or RANKL (RANK Ligand). RANKL is secreted by osteoblast (bone building) cells once the cells have completed their cycle of bone building. The drug binds to RANKL and inhibits or slows down the effects of RANKL, thereby slowing down the tearing down of bone.*

- *Multiple mechanisms of action at work are drugs where the MOA is unclear, but the actions of more than one mechanism combine to produce a positive impact on bone.*

## ROUTE OF ADMINISTRATION

Most drugs can be administered into the body through different routes, including: nasal spray (daily); taking oral pills (daily, weekly or monthly); infusions or intravenous therapy (every three weeks or once yearly); or subcutaneous (just below the skin) injections (once daily or every six months). Not all drugs are available in all forms. Work with your healthcare provider to find the drug that is most effective and affordable for you and best suits your lifestyle. Research shows that people are more likely to take their medication as prescribed if they have agreed to the route and frequency of administration.

Before prescribing a drug therapy, your doctor will consider factors such as your genetics, medical history and lifestyle to identify which drug action would likely be the best for you.

## BENEFIT, RISK AND COST FACTORS

Before going on a medication for osteoporosis, consider the degree of benefit together with its risks and cost. Consider your risk assessment results for both osteoporosis and fracture. Individuals assessed as having normal or low risk can often manage the disease through a healthy lifestyle with adequate intake of calcium, vitamin D and appropriate exercise. They do not usually require a medication therapy at this point in time. Individuals assessed as moderate risk of osteoporosis and fracture should discuss, with their doctor, the risks and benefits of taking or not taking a medication based on medical status, age and fracture risk over the next 10 years. For individuals assessed as high risk or who have had a low trauma fracture, there is evidence that osteoporosis medication will be of significant benefit to them. In all cases, the decision to take medication is yours.

For example, most experts agree that alendronate, risedronate and zoledronic acid are among the most effective bisphosphonates for reducing fractures. If your 10-year fracture risk is 18 percent (moderate risk), therapy for 10 years would reduce your fracture risk to about nine percent (low risk). If you had an annual fracture risk of two percent (low risk), your annual fracture risk would be reduced to one percent (low risk) with bisphosphonate therapy.

You can see where people with a greater risk of fracture have the greatest gain or benefit. When deciding whether to start a medication, determine the degree of benefit, the risk and severity of side effects and the cost prior to making your decision.

## SIDE EFFECTS AND RARE EVENTS

Side effects and rare events may occur when taking any drug. Side effects are commonly linked with drugs. Side effects tend to be mild, usually go away in a few days and do not cause long-term damage. Keep all side effects in perspective. Most side effects go away with time; others may be recurrent.

Some side effects can be eliminated by taking precautions to avoid anything that may make you more susceptible to that side effect. For example, side effects related to the IV infusion of zoledronic acid can be minimized by drinking plenty of fluids during the day of infusion, particularly right after the infusion is completed.

Rare events are more serious, but less common. There is always a risk that a devastating, but rare event may occur from taking any drug. Unfortunately, it is not possible to predict when a rare event will occur or who it will affect. Even common, everyday foods have a rare event risk. For example, some people have life-threatening allergic reactions to peanuts or seafood. However, not everyone knows they are allergic. Unless a person has been diagnosed with a specific allergy and knows its effect, that person's reaction to consuming these foods would be unpredictable as would a rare event from taking a drug. Be sure to discuss the significance of any side effects you encounter with your doctor or pharmacist.

Results from clinical studies provide some information of what to expect when taking a drug. The frequency of side effects that occur when subjects are treated with the study drug compared to a placebo (sugar pill) gives some idea of the chances of experiencing some of the common side effects (see Chapter 12).

Examine the potential positive and negative results of taking any drug to prevent or treat your osteoporosis. Look at the unchanged course of the disease should you choose not to take the drug. Consider your risk of fracture or breaking a bone and how this might affect your quality of life. After doing your own research and discussing this with your doctor, ask yourself: "Do the benefits of taking or not taking a drug outweigh the short-term and long-term risks of fracture?"

## TREATMENTS FOR OSTEOPOROSIS

- *Bisphosphonates*
- *SERMs (Estrogen Agonist, Antagonist)*
- *RANK Ligand Inhibitors*
- *Calcitonin*
- *Parathyroid Hormone*
- *Hormone Therapy (HT)*

About 50% of women who start taking a drug therapy for osteoporosis will discontinue it within one year and the majority should not stop.

### Bisphosphonates

Bisphosphonates are a non-hormonal group of drugs that fall under the category of anti-resorptive drug. Since the 1970s, bisphosphonates have been used to treat other bone disorders, such as Paget's disease, where there is excessive breakdown and formation of bone resulting in weak bone and fractures. Since the 1990s, bisphosphonates have been used to treat osteoporosis in women and men.

Bisphosphonates have a common basic chemical structure made up of phosphonates, oxygen atoms and carbon atoms. As other groups of atoms are added, a new bisphosphonate is created. Bisphosphonates vary depending on what combination of atoms is placed in which location. Because bisphosphonates have slightly differing characteristics, one bisphosphonate may be more effective than another for a particular therapy.

When searching the internet, you may find bisphosphonates that are not available in your country. Approved bisphosphonates available in the United States and Canada are alendronate (Fosamax, Fosavance), risedronate (Actonel, Actonel with Calcium, Atelvia) and zoledronic acid (Reclast, Aclasta). The United States also has ibandronate (Boniva) while Canada has etidronate (Didrocal). While other bisphosphonates are available in the United States and Canada, they have not been approved for use in osteoporosis by the FDA or TPD.

### BENEFITS OF BISPHOSPHONATES
Alendronate (Fosamax, Fosavance), available since the mid 1990s, and Risedronate (Actonel, Actonel with Calcium, Atelvia), available since the late 1990s, both:

- *More potent than etidronate*

- *Approved for prevention and treatment of osteoporosis*

- *Approved for use in post-menopausal women, glucocorticoid-induced osteoporosis, and osteoporosis in men*

- *Build bone density in the spine and hip*

- *Reduce fractures in the spine and hip*

Zoledronic acid (Reclast, Aclasta) approved in North America in 2007:

- *More potent than etidronate*

- *Approved for prevention and treatment of osteoporosis*

- *Approved for use in post-menopausal women, glucocorticoid-induced osteoporosis, and osteoporosis in men*

- *Builds bone density in the spine and hip*

- *Reduces fractures in the spine and hip*

- *Administered once a year by intravenous infusion*

- *Has shown a 40 percent decrease in risk of hip fracture in women 65 to 89 years of age*

Ibandronate (Boniva) available in the United States:

- *More potent than etidronate*
- *Approved for prevention and treatment of osteoporosis*
- *Reduces the incidence of spine fractures*

Etidronate (Didrocal), a less potent drug, used for osteoporosis:

- *Reduces spinal fractures when taken with calcium (calcium is not be taken on the same day as etidronate)*

Clodronate and IV pamidronate are bisphosphonates that are not widely studied and have not been approved as osteoporosis therapies.

Do not take bisphosphonates if you have hypocalcemia (low levels of calcium in the blood) and have impaired kidney function. If you are unable to swallow or remain upright after taking a medication, do not take oral dosages. When taking any osteoporosis drug, make sure you also take the optimum amount of calcium and vitamin D. Calcium cannot be taken at the same time as a bisphosphonate.

### ROUTE OF ADMINISTRATION FOR BISPHOSPHONATES

When taking an oral bisphosphonate, there are some important rules to remember so that the drug is most effective and has minimal side effects.

- *Rule 1: Do not have calcium two hours before or after. If you take calcium supplements while also taking oral bisphosphonates, make sure you take the calcium at least two hours before or two hours after the bisphosphonate. If the bisphosphonate comes in contact with calcium, it will bind to the calcium and make the drug inactive.*

- *Rule 2: Take whole with plain water. Tablets should not be broken, crushed or chewed. Bisphosphonates can cause an irritation in the esophagus (the food pipe). They should be taken whole with at least one-half to one glass of plain water. The water ensures delivery of the tablet to the stomach as quickly as possible without causing any esophageal side effects. Some tablets have a special coating to help them move quickly to the stomach.*

- *Rule 3: Take with water on an empty stomach first thing in the morning and do not eat for at least 30 minutes. Medications, food and beverages other than plain water can all interfere with the absorption of orally-administered bisphosphonates, except with delayed-release risedronate (Atelvia) taken immediately after breakfast. They may bind together and inactivate the bisphosphonate so it does not work. Waiting 60 minutes may work even better.*

- *Rule 4: Remain upright, either sitting or standing for 30 minutes after. Do not lie down for at least 30 minutes and until after eating your first food of the day. This will help protect your esophagus (food pipe) from unnecessary irritation or burning.*

Alendronate (Fosamax, Fosavance), either as a tablet or liquid, is taken daily or weekly. A combined version of alendronate with 2,800IU or 5,600IU of vitamin D, known as Fosavance, is taken once weekly.

Risedronate (Actonel, Actonel with Calcium) offers some flexibility. In addition to daily or weekly dosing, it is available in a monthly dosing tablet. A version is also available as a combined package that has both risedronate and calcium. Each week of therapy consists of seven tablets, one taken each day for a week (one Actonel 35mg tablet and six calcium carbonate 1250mg tablets). In addition, a delayed-release version of risedronate (Atlevia) can be taken immediately after breakfast.

Zoledronic acid (Reclast, Aclasta) is given once yearly via an infusion (intravenously in the arm). To minimize side effects, be sure to be well hydrated by drinking lots of fluids the morning prior to the infusion. Drink at least two quarts or liters of fluids during the day of the infusion and at least two glasses (16oz/500ml) of water after the infusion.

Ibandronate (Boniva), which is available in the United States, can be administered either as a tablet or intravenously. Tablets are taken as a daily or monthly regimen in the morning. Intravenous (IV) injections are administered once every three months.

Available in some countries, etidronate and calcium (Didrocal) is a combination medication that is administered in a 90-day cycle. Each cycle consists of 14 days of taking only etidronate tablets (400mg per dose), then 76 days of taking only calcium carbonate tablets (500mg per dose). The etidronate tablets are taken on an empty stomach with a full glass of water (8oz/250ml) at least two hours away from other foods, drinks or medications. The calcium carbonate may be taken with or without food, but preferably with food, to help maximize the absorption of calcium. After 90 days, the cycle is repeated. Unlike other bisphosphonates that are usually taken in the morning, etidronate can be taken at other times of the day, even just prior to bedtime.

The use of bisphosphonates in pre-menopausal women (during childbearing years) has not been studied, so there are significant concerns about the use of bisphosphonates in women who may get pregnant. Since bisphosphonates may remain in bone for many years because of the slow release, there may be adverse effects on the normal bone development of a fetus, baby or child. If you are pre-menopausal and have osteoporosis, discuss treatment options with your doctor, including the risks and benefits of each treatment.

If at any time you are unclear about your medication, check with your doctor or pharmacist to make sure you are taking the medication correctly.

### SIDE EFFECTS OF BISPHOSPHONATES

Oral bisphosphonates are generally well tolerated when taken properly. However, there can be side effects of bisphosphonates, which include:

When deciding to take a drug, consider the benefits and risks associated with your individual health status.

- *Nausea*

- *Heartburn*

- *Constipation or diarrhea*

- *Abdominal pain*

- *Bone and joint pain all over*

- *Esophageal burning (rare, but make sure you take it with enough water).*

Some rare side effects associated with bisphosphonates are discussed below to help you understand what can be done to minimize the risk of occurrence.

### ESOPHAGEAL ULCER

Some degree of heartburn may be associated with bisphosphonates. If the heartburn is persistent or severe, you should advise your doctor. The medication may have to be discontinued and further investigation done to determine if you have an esophageal ulcer. To avoid this complication, do not lie down until after you have had something to eat no earlier than 30 minutes after taking the bisphosphonate (60 minutes in the case of ibandronate). Some experts feel the risk is lower when the brand-name version of the bisphosphonate is taken as opposed to a generic version because of differences in the tablet shape and/or coating. Be sure to follow the instructions for drinking enough water. If you have been told you have any abnormality in the esophagus, you should speak with your doctor before taking a bisphosphonate.

### OSTEONECROSIS OF THE JAW

Several years ago, osteonecrosis of the jaw (ONJ) was reported in the media as a devastating condition occurring with the use of bisphosphonates. Many people stopped their medication without good reason. This unpredictable and rare event was mainly associated with the use of intravenous bisphosphonates given at higher doses and for treatment in patients with cancer and not osteoporosis.

Osteonecrosis of the jaw shows up as an area of exposed bone inside the mouth that may or may not be painful. Among people who have developed osteonecrosis of the jaw, it has been observed that 50 percent had recent dental procedures. The strongest association is in patients with cancer (breast, prostate, myeloma) who have been on monthly intravenous bisphosphonates for a year or longer. It is important to point out that one study of more than 7,000 post-menopausal women with osteoporosis showed that the occurrence of osteonecrosis of the jaw was the same whether they received intravenous bisphosphonates or not. Only one patient in each group developed osteonecrosis of the jaw.

Some dentists do not feel comfortable performing dental work on a person who is taking a bisphosphonate. Some bone experts and some dentists recommend delaying the start of the bisphosphonate therapy until after major dental work has been completed or stopping the bisphosphonate for up to three months prior to major or significant dental procedures, such as tooth extractions or dental implants. Other more common dental procedures, such as root canals or scaling, do not pose the same concerns for these experts and dentists. There are no recognized studies that prove these recommendations to be effective methods in reducing the possible risk of osteonecrosis of the jaw. This is a situation that should be discussed with your doctor and dentist to identify your risks and benefits of the different options.

### ATRIAL FIBRILLATION

The human heart normally beats at a regular, steady pace or rate. Atrial fibrillation is an irregular beating of a small chamber of the heart. Atrial fibrillation is a common form of irregular heart beat that increases in frequency with age and has been reported, coincidentally, with bisphosphonate use. It is unclear from the medical literature whether it is truly caused by bisphosphonate use. Most experts do not feel this is of significant concern and some feel that there may be people who might be at a unique risk for this problem. This area is undergoing active research.

## FRACTURE BENEFIT AND DELIVERY METHOD FOR BISPHOSPHONATES

| | Studies show decrease in fractures of the spine at 3 years | Studies show decrease in fractures of the hip at 3 years | Delivery Method |
|---|---|---|---|
| Alendronate (Fosamax, Fosavance) | Extremely effective | Mildly effective | Tablets daily or weekly |
| Risedronate (Actonel, Actonel with Calcium) | Extremely effective | Mildly effective | Tablets daily, weekly or monthly |
| Zoledronic acid (Reclast, Aclasta) | Extremely effective | Moderately effective | Intravenous every 12 months |
| Ibandronate (Boniva) | Extremely effective | Insufficient data | Tablets daily or monthly, or intravenous every three months |
| Etidronate (Didrocal) | Moderately effective | Insufficient data | Tablets 14 days and calcium 76 days |

### ATYPICAL FRACTURES (CHALK STICK FRACTURE)

There have been some reports of individuals who have been on a bisphosphonate for many years and developed unusual fractures of the femur (upper leg bone), known as an atypical fracture. This fracture occurs rarely. Many of these patients report having had the pain in their thigh or groin region for some time before the fracture occurs. Little is known about why this fracture occurs. It has been associated with long-term use of a bisphosphonate (usually five years or longer), but it is difficult to identify its cause and what precautions can be taken. Some experts feel this rare occurrence may be due to bisphosphonates slowing and interfering with the remodeling process in certain bones. People who have never been on a bisphosphonate have also experienced this type of fracture.

Atypical fractures are sometimes referred to as "chalk stick fractures" because breaks occur straight across the bone. As atypical fractures are very rare and as bisphosphonates typically prevent fractures from occurring, experts suggest that if you experience new pain in your leg or hip region lasting for several days, talk with your doctor about your symptoms.

## SERMs (Selective Estrogen Receptor Modulators)

Historically, tamoxifen (Nolvadex, Tamofen) is a selective estrogen receptor modulator (SERM) that has been used for many years to slow and prevent the recurrence of breast cancer in post-menopausal women. Experts treating breast cancer initially thought tamoxifen might block the effect of estrogen and result in increased bone loss. Studies noted that bone density in women on tamoxifen increased over a few years. This observation led to bone health studies with other SERMs, such as raloxifene (Evista).

SERMs work as an anti-resorptive on bone for women. SERMs are not estrogens; they are a compound that interacts with the body's tissues. Sometimes the SERM acts like estrogen (agonist) and, at other times, it has the effect of blocking estrogen (antagonist). These different SERMs may have different effects on estrogen dependent tissues and are, therefore, said to be selective. For example, it has been reported that whereas tamoxifen has some effect on the endometrium (lining of the uterus) and may be associated with a slight risk of endometrial or uterine cancer, raloxifene does not have any effect on the endometrium and does not appear to increase the risk of endometrial or uterine cancer. As well, this selective action is very encouraging news for women who are at risk of osteoporosis, but will not or cannot take estrogen therapy.

### BENEFITS OF SERMS

- *Slows the rate of rapid bone turnover in post-menopausal women to that of pre-menopausal women*

- *Stabilizes bone density and reduces fractures of the spine*

- *Improves lipid profile by reducing LDL (bad cholesterol) and total cholesterol (the overall impact on cardiovascular risk requires further study).*

- *Reduces risk of invasive breast cancer in women at risk of invasive breast cancer*

- *No increase in endometrial cancer or endometrial thickness, so no breakthrough bleeding*

- *Simple and easy to take any time of day with or without food*

Raloxifene has been approved in North America for use by otherwise healthy post-menopausal women to prevent and treat osteoporosis. Most experts find that SERMs are most appropriate for active women in their sixties as they have been shown to reduce spine fracture risk. However, SERMs have not been shown to reduce the risk of hip or other fractures. Therefore, they are not typically used in treatments for the very elderly.

In the United States, raloxifene has also been approved for use in reducing the risk of invasive breast cancer in post-menopausal women with osteoporosis or who are at high risk for invasive breast cancer.

### ROUTE OF ADMINISTRATION OF SERMS
Raloxifene is taken daily as a single dose medication and can be taken with or without food. For people who experience stomach upset from taking raloxifene, taking it with meals may help to reduce or eliminate the discomfort.

### SIDE EFFECTS OF SERMS
- *Hot flashes, particularly in women under 60*
- *Leg cramps or leg swelling*
- *Deep vein thrombosis (blood clots)*
- *Joint pain*
- *Flu-like symptoms (fever, cough, body aches).*

A word of caution, post-menopausal symptoms, such as hot flashes (flushes) and other vasomotor symptoms, are not effectively managed by SERMs and may in fact get worse. One of the side effects of raloxifene/SERMs is deep vein thrombosis, which is also associated with estrogen therapy. Raloxifene/SERMs should not be taken by women with liver problems, who are or may become pregnant, or who are at increased risk for stroke or blood clots. This includes women who have had previous strokes, blood clots, transient ischemic attacks (TIAs), atrial fibrillation or uncontrolled high blood pressure. Be sure to check with your doctor.

**FRACTURE BENEFIT AND DELIVERY METHOD FOR SERMS**

| | Studies show decrease in fractures of the spine at 3 years | Studies show decrease in fractures of the hip at 3 years | Delivery Method |
|---|---|---|---|
| **Raloxifene (Evista)** | Extremely effective | Insufficient data | Pills daily |

## RANK Ligand Inhibitors

Denosumab (Prolia) is a RANK Ligand inhibitor that has a more direct effect than other anti-resorptive drugs on the bone remodeling process. Denosumab is a protein that has specific binding targets. The mechanism of action for denosumab is unique in that it effects the action of RANKL directly and interferes with the RANKL pathway. It does this by acting like the protein osteoprotegerin (OPG). In Chapter 1 we discussed how OPG slows down bone loss.

*Drugs can interfere with the action of the protein RANKL, thereby slowing down the tearing down of bone.*

Denosumab has effects like an anti-resorptive. It interferes with the RANKL's normal actions of stimulating osteoclast cells increasing bone resorption. It does this by binding to the RANKL and inhibiting stimulation and, therefore, the growth of the osteoclasts. This action mimics the effects of the body's natural defense mechanism of using OPG, which slows down bone removal. Studies suggest denosumab may be more efficient at stopping osteoclasts than some other currently available therapies.

### BENEFITS OF RANKL INHIBITORS

- *Shown to decrease spinal, hip and other fractures*

- *Increases bone density to a larger amount than other anti-resorptives. A reduction in spinal fractures was noticed at one year after the start of therapy. With other anti-resorptives, bone density typically increases over three years, but slows down by the third year. With denosumab, the rate of increase does not seem to slow at three years. The significance of this is still under study.*

### ROUTE OF ADMINISTRATION OF RANKL INHIBITORS

Denosumab is administered by subcutaneous injection every six months for the treatment of osteoporosis. Injections can be done simply by you at home after receiving guidance and education on the technique. It is the same method used for insulin injections in patients with diabetes. Since the injection is given only twice a year, you could also ask your doctor, nurse or qualified pharmacist to provide the injection.

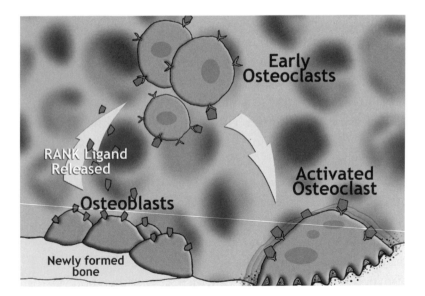

- *Rash*

- *Infection*

- *Headache*

- *Constipation*

- *Sore throat*

- *Joint pain*

Denosumab is a biologically derived drug treatment (made using living cells and processes rather than chemical reactions). This treatment has not shown to be associated with an increased risk of cancer and cardiovascular disease, although there is still some concern that it may. Other concerns are delayed fracture healing, hypocalcemia, osteonecrosis of the jaw or atypical fractures. Not all biologic treatments share the same side effects or mechanism of action. As with all potential side effects, they should be considered in relation to overall benefits of the treatment. Talk with your doctor and pharmacist about the drug and your medical history. Discuss the benefits of the treatment versus the risk of any possible side effect or rare event.

**FRACTURE BENEFIT AND DELIVERY METHOD FOR DENOSUMAB**

| | Studies show decrease in fractures of the spine at 3 years | Studies show decrease in fractures of the hip at 3 years | Delivery Method |
|---|---|---|---|
| Denosumab (Prolia) | Extremely effective | Moderately effective | Injection below the skin every 6 months |

## Calcitonin

Calcitonin has been approved in the United States and Canada and other countries for the treatment of osteoporosis. Approved for use in women at least five years beyond menopause, calcitonin treatment may be considered for men or women when bisphosphonates cannot be taken and other osteoporosis therapies have been considered.

### BENEFITS OF CALCITONIN

Calcitonin works as an anti-resorptive. It is a natural human hormone involved in calcium regulation and bone metabolism. Some of its benefits are similar to estrogen and bisphosphonates. Calcitonin reduces bone loss by inhibiting the osteoclasts (reducing bone breakdown). It has been shown that, in the first few years of treatment, calcitonin slightly increases bone density in the spine. Furthermore, calcitonin has no affect on other tissues, such as breast tissue, the uterus or the heart.

Calcitonin has been found to decrease acute pain caused by fractures of the spine. The exact mechanism of how calcitonin provides an analgesic (pain relieving) effect to fracture pain is not known. Pain relief from use of calcitonin is not usually immediate. Taking normal dosages of nasal spray calcitonin may or may not be effective in reducing pain associated with a fracture. If your doctor recommends that you use calcitonin to reduce pain, you may need to take a large dose by injection. It may take up to a few days before you experience any pain relief.

A five-year study with nasal spray calcitonin at 200IU per day showed a reduction in spinal fractures. However, further research, including administering a higher dose, did not confirm this benefit. There is controversy of how the study was conducted and some experts feel that the results are not reliable.

### ROUTE OF ADMINISTRATION OF CALCITONIN

Calcitonin is available as a nasal spray (Miacalcin, Fortical) or injection (Calcimar, Miacalcin) under the skin using a needle similar to giving insulin or injected into the muscle (intermuscular). Nasal spray salmon calcitonin is convenient to use at any time of day regardless of meals or medications. It can be safely used with all other medications. Salmon calcitonin (calcitonin derived from the fish salmon) should be kept in the refrigerator until the bottle is opened. Once opened, the drug can be stored for up to 35 days at room temperature.

### SIDE EFFECTS OF CALCITONIN

- *Nasal spray calcitonin may result in nasal congestion (usually minor)*
- *Flushing of the hands and feet*
- *Frequent urination*
- *Light-headedness*
- *Skin rash*
- *Nausea, vomiting and diarrhea (rare)*
- *Allergic reaction (rare, but can be very serious)*

### FRACTURE BENEFIT AND DELIVERY METHOD FOR CALCITONIN

| | Studies show decrease in fractures of the spine at 3 years | Studies show decrease in fractures of the hip at 3 years | Delivery Method |
|---|---|---|---|
| Calcitonin (Miacalcin, Fortical, Calcimar) | Mild to moderately effective | No data | Nasal spray daily or injections under the skin |

## Parathyroid Hormone

Teriparatide (Forteo) is a synthetic or artificial form of the naturally occurring parathyroid hormone (PTH). It is a relatively new osteoporosis treatment that directly impacts the bone building or the anabolic part of the bone remodeling process. Teriparatide is approved for treatment in post-menopausal women, for men at high risk for fracture and for glucocorticoid-induced osteoporosis. It has been shown in studies to reduce spinal fractures and other fractures (not including hip fractures) compared to a placebo over 18 months. Teriparatide is currently the only approved anabolic agent for the treatment of osteoporosis available in North America.

### BENEFITS OF PARATHYROID HORMONE

Parathyroid hormone is a naturally occurring hormone that regulates serum calcium (calcium found in blood). Too much parathyroid hormone on a continuous basis, known as hyperparathyroidism, can cause osteoporosis and fractures. However, when parathyroid hormone is given as a single daily injection, it has been shown to be a potent agent that can stimulate osteoblasts and bone formation. In contrast to anti-resorptive drugs, parathyroid hormone leads to forming new bone and not just preventing the loss of existing bone

Clinical studies using parathyroid hormone injections in humans have shown significant increases in bone density. Bone formed with parathyroid hormone therapy is of normal quality and strength.

### ROUTE OF ADMINISTRATION OF PARATHYROID HORMONE

Parathyroid hormone is taken as a daily subcutaneous (below the skin) injection, usually in the thigh or abdomen. It is recommended for use for up to 24 months, at which time your doctor would switch you to a different therapy, likely an anti-resorptive agent. Other parathyroid hormone preparations are in development or available in Europe.

### SIDE EFFECTS OF PARATHYROID HORMONE

- *Headache*
- *Dizziness*
- *Nausea*
- *Leg cramps*
- *Reactions at the injection site*

### POSSIBLE CONCERNS OF PARATHYROID HORMONE

Hypercalcemia (increased blood levels of calcium) is rare and total calcium intake should be less than 1,200mg per day. Vitamin D should be limited to about 1,000IU per day. As well, your doctor will monitor you closely if you have a history of gout.

## CONTRAINDICATIONS (REASONS NOT TO USE THE THERAPY)

People with the following should not use PTH:

- *Severe kidney problems*

- *Bone cancer*

- *Primary hyperparathyroidism*

- *Paget's disease*

- *Pregnant*

- *Under radiation therapy involving the skeleton or for bone cancer*

- *Growing skeletons (young children)*

The risk of osteosarcoma (bone cancer) with teriparatide use has been associated with studies in laboratory rats, but not in humans. Most experts feel the findings from these studies do not translate into humans. The safety and benefits of teriparatide have not been evaluated beyond two years. As a safety measure and until further research is completed, the duration for use of teriparatide is limited to 24 months.

### FRACTURE BENEFIT AND DELIVERY METHOD FOR PARATHYROID HORMONE

| | Studies show decrease in fractures of the spine at 3 years | Studies show decrease in fractures of the hip at 3 years | Delivery Method |
|---|---|---|---|
| Teriparatide (Forteo) | Extremely effective | Insufficient data | Daily injection under the skin |

## Estrogen and Progesterone Therapy for Women

Hormone therapy used to be the first treatment considered for the prevention or treatment of osteoporosis in women younger than 65. With the advent of other drug therapies, estrogen has been taken off the primary list of osteoporosis treatments in the United States and is considered second-line therapy in Canada. Prevention of bone loss is now considered an unintentional benefit when using hormone therapy to treat peri-menopausal symptoms. The widely publicized Women's Health Initiative study showed that hormone therapy reduced the risk of fractures, particularly hip fractures. However, some serious risks were increased (see Chapter 2). Although hormone therapy is sometimes used for prevention of osteoporosis, it is unlikely that it will be used for treatment of osteoporosis unless severe menopausal symptoms are also an issue.

## Testosterone Replacement Therapy for Men

Testosterone replacement therapy has both anti-resorptive and anabolic properties. It is meant as a preventive measure for osteoporosis when indicated for men who generally display other hypogonadal symptoms. It is not considered a medical treatment for osteoporosis as there are more effective medical treatments available for bone loss.

As noted in Chapter 3, some experts have concerns about using testosterone replacement therapy due to its possible effect on the prostate gland. This is similar to the issue of estrogen and breast cancer in women. The risk of testosterone replacement therapy should be considered on an individual basis. Remember to establish your personal fracture risk based on your medical history, risk of hypogonadal symptoms and risk of a fracture.

## Strontium Ranelate

(Not available in North America)
Strontium ranelate is a salt agent thought to have a mechanism of action that stimulates bone formation and decreases bone breakdown. Strontium ranelate (Protelos, Protos) is not available in North America, but is being used in Europe, Asia and Australia. Studies have shown that, as an osteoporosis therapy, strontium ranelate reduces vertebral, hip and other fractures.

Health food stores and natural health product stores may sell other types of strontium salts such as strontium chloride, citrate and gluconate. Strontium salts other than ranelate are not proven to reduce fractures, and side effects of the non-ranelate salts are not well documented. The main issues with these non-ranelate strontium salts include the low dose of strontium contained in each pill and the lack of evidence that these other salts have a beneficial effect on bones. Be aware that not all strontium salts have the same effects on the body or bone.

### ROUTE OF ADMINISTRATION STRONTIUM RANELATE
Strontium ranelate comes as small packets of powder that is mixed with water and taken orally daily. It is best taken two hours after a meal and preferably at bedtime.

### SIDE EFFECTS STRONTIUM RANELATE

- *Headache*

- *Nausea*

- *Diarrhea*

Strontium ranelate is generally well tolerated and side effects are usually not serious.

*Education and a good relationship with your healthcare providers can improve your treatment outcome.*

## Tibolone

**(Not available in North America)**
Currently available in Europe, tibolone (Livial) has combined progesterone, estrogen and testosterone properties that offer a positive alternative treatment for post-menopausal symptoms and to prevent osteoporosis in women. It may also improve libido (sexual desire) in women. It is not available in North America, although it has been used for decades in Europe. The side effects of this drug have not been well studied.

# CANCER MEDICATIONS AND GLUCOCORTICOIDS: TREATMENTS TO PROTECT BONE

## Treatment for Patients on Glucocorticoids

Prednisone doses as low as 2.5mg a day have a small effect in contributing to bone loss and osteoporosis. At higher doses of 5mg a day or more, there is a twofold increase of fractures of the spine and hip. Inhaled steroids have a slight effect on bone. Generally, inhaled steroids are more topical (to the respiratory lining) and have a less systemic effect. However, high doses of potent inhaled steroids will have a slight effect and if given with intermittent oral prednisone, increased bone loss effect could be significant.

Patients need to maintain a healthy lifestyle that includes good calcium and vitamin D intake and regular physical exercise. In patients with fractures or significant bone loss, treatments to slow resorption (bisphosphonates, calcitonin, estrogen, testosterone, denosumab) should be considered. If there is marked bone loss and a significant concern about fractures, a bone formation medication, such as parathyroid hormone, may be required.

## Treatment for Women on Cancer Medication

Female patients with breast cancer should be offered treatment for osteoporosis if they have established fractures and/or low bone density. Patients who are estrogen receptor positive may be considered for ovarian resection if pre-menopausal. Post-menopausal patients may be offered treatment with a selective estrogen receptor modulator (tamoxifen, raloxifene) or an aromatase inhibitor. SERMs slow and prevent the recurrence of breast cancer in post-menopausal women and stabilize bone density. Bisphosphonates, taken orally or intravenously, have a favorable effect even if the patient is estrogen deficient. Other therapies, including denosumab or parathyroid hormone, may also have a role in treating women with cancer.

## Treatment for Men on Cancer Medication

Men who have undergone treatment for local or advanced prostate cancer may be at increased risk for osteoporosis. Targeted therapies involving surgery or radiotherapy may further include adjuvant therapies that decrease serum testosterone levels. Testosterone deficiency may cause an accelerated loss of bone resulting in osteoporosis.

Therapy should include lifestyle recommendations (calcium, vitamin D and physical activity), and may include therapies such as bisphosphonates, denosumab or parathyroid hormone. Treatment decisions should be based on bone density, the severity of bone loss and the presence or absence of fractures. Life expectancy may or may not be important in the treatment decision.

Men who have experienced the spread of cancer to the bone may be advised to have monthly treatment with an intravenous bisphosphonate, such as zolendronic acid (Zometa, Aclasta, Reclast).

## FUTURE DRUG THERAPIES

The future of osteoporosis therapy looks promising. Here are some of the drug therapies that are in the early stages of development:

- *Odanacatib is a cathepsin K inhibitor. Cathepsin K is an enzyme that plays an essential role in the function of osteoclasts and the breakdown of bone.*

- *Apomine is a bisphosphonate ester that has stimulated new bone formation in animal studies.*

- *Oral calcitonin is a convenient and reliable form of calcitonin for osteoporosis treatment.*

- *Bazedoxifene and Lasofoxifene are SERMs with a variation in the amount of estrogen receptor modulating activity leading to a refinement of SERM effects. Lasofoxifene has been approved for use in Europe.*

- *Ronacaleret is a calcilytic that blocks the parathyroid calcium sensing receptor leading to the body's pulse of parathyroid hormone that triggers bone building properties. The result is bursts of parathyroid hormone that stimulates osteoblasts.*

- *Sclerostin antibody is an agent that binds and inhibits sclerostin, a protein that blocks or slows bone formation.*

- *Menatetrenone is a vitamin K derivative that may inhibit osteoclasts as well as help with the normalization of mineralizing (hardening) of bone.*

## Vertebroplasty and Kyphoplasty

At some point you may hear about vertebroplasty or kyphoplasty – procedures to stabilize vertebral fractures, which are a common result of osteoporosis. Although not yet well researched for use in treating osteoporosis, these procedures are offered by some doctors to improve symptoms, such as pain, that may be associated with fractures from osteoporosis. However, they are not a treatment for osteoporosis or to strengthen the spine. Even if you have these procedures, you will still need to receive a drug therapy for osteoporosis.

Vertebroplasty involves injecting bone cement mixture through a long needle into the fractured vertebra, filling the spaces within the bone. The needle is removed and the cement hardens.

In kyphoplasty, a balloon is inserted through a long needle into the vertebra and gently inflated to create a cavity or space. The balloon is then removed and bone cement is injected into the space where it hardens.

The procedure to inject cement into bone was initially developed for patients who had multiple myeloma or bone marrow cancer. It was shown to be very successful in preventing collapse of the spine. The procedure to inject cement is usually performed by radiologists or surgeons in people who have fractures of the spine from osteoporosis.

Laughter boosts the immune system and reduces pain by releasing endorphins that are more potent than equivalent amounts of morphine.

The average kindergarten student laughs 300 times a day, an adult laughs just 17 times a day. Laughter dissolves tension, stress, anxiety, depression and anger.

Although it has become increasingly popular, there have only been limited studies to show that this procedure has merit. In two small studies, patients who had this procedure did no better than if they did not have the procedure. Radiologists who do this procedure say the studies were too small to show benefit. However, it should be pointed out that if there is a benefit, it is likely a small benefit for a select group of patients. One concern to be aware of is the slight increased risk of fracture above and below the level of the procedure.

Vertebroplasty and kyphoplasty are most suited for people who have chronic pain due to spinal fractures. You may wish to discuss these procedures with your doctor.

# CHAPTER 11 KEY POINTS

- The goal of drug therapy is to reduce fracture risk by preventing further bone loss and promoting strong bones.

- Drugs work in different ways to produce an effect on the body and improve bone density.

- Drugs can: slow down osteoclasts or bone removal cells; speed up osteoblasts or bone formation cells; interfere with the action of the protein RANKL, thereby slowing down the tearing down of bone; have an unclear action of more than one mechanism.

- When deciding to take a drug, consider the benefits and risks associated with your individual health status, lifestyle preferences and your risk of osteoporosis and risk of fracture.

- Look at the unchanged course of the disease should you choose not to take the drug.

- Keep side effects in perspective. Most go away with time; others may be recurrent. Take steps to minimize the occurrence of side effects.

- Rare events can be more serious, but less common.

- Be sure to check with your doctor on how best to protect your bones if you are on cancer medication or glucocorticoids (prednisone).

# Understanding Health Headlines

The internet is full of useful information. It is also full of information that, if not fully understood, can be misinterpreted. Today's patient has a great opportunity to be more informed about his or her condition and the possible treatments, simply by getting information from the internet. The temptation for many, however, is to present this information to their doctor to "sort out" for them or to determine their own treatment.

Learning is a powerful tool, but only if we understand and apply what we learn. We are constantly being exposed to reports and medical studies that tell us something will affect our health in one way or another. It is important to evaluate the credibility of what is being said and how it applies to your personal health situation.

Health choices should be based on valid evidence from scientific research. Major scientific medical journals have a process called "peer-review" that helps to ensure that the research being reported is valid and unbiased. Once research is published, healthcare professionals can read, assess and discuss the value of the findings with colleagues in order to determine whether this information will apply to their own practice and ultimately benefit their patients.

## BE CAUTIOUS WHEN READING HEADLINES

News headlines are supposed to grab our attention, which sometimes causes unnecessary concern.

**"Calcium pills raise heart risk" (BBC)**

**"New Zealand research has found that older women taking calcium to protect their bones had a higher risk of heart attack" (ABC)**

**"Calcium supplements raise heart-attack risk: Study" (CTV)**

These headlines resulted from the publication of a study in the *BMJ* (British Medical Journal), a well known and reputable international peer reviewed medical journal. The New Zealand study, which we first referred to in Chapter 4, compared a relatively small group of women taking calcium supplements to the same number of women taking a placebo (sugar pills). Calcium citrate was used to provide 1,000mg of elemental calcium daily for those taking the active treatment. What was surprising, and was not mentioned in the news broadcasts, was that these women on average consumed 860mg of dietary calcium in addition to the 1,000mg supplement. The average North American intake of dietary calcium is usually less than 700mg daily.

Many of the news broadcasts reporting on this study did not report that other studies amounting to more than 30,000 participants have been done before. These studies did not show calcium to negatively affect the cardiovascular (heart and blood vessels) system. Some indicated calcium may in fact be beneficial. The New Zealand study was designed to see if calcium would have beneficial effects on the cardiovascular system. It is possible that the cardiovascular risks were just due to chance rather than the increased calcium intake, but the study design did not gather that information.

The Women's Health Initiative, a major reputable study, which we referred to in Chapters 2 and 4, did not confirm a link between calcium supplements and increased heart complications.

While research is ongoing to determine the optimal amount of daily calcium we should have, media and consumers have access to scientific information and published articles on the various studies. Given the restrictions of air time or print space, the reporting of medical information in the media can be a challenge. Media organizations select what they feel the public should know and are often accused of being sensational in their reporting. It is up to consumers to seek out more detail about what they have heard or read. It is necessary to separate what was implied only to make a headline and what was pure fact from the study. Checking with your doctor is a good place to start before making changes to your treatment or care plan.

As a patient, you should maintain an interest and be involved in the choice of treatment prescribed for you. Keep up on recent developments that may apply to your care. Do your own research and be prepared to discuss new treatment options and your alternatives with your doctor. The reason you are seeking out a doctor's care is ultimately for his or her professional experience and judgment to help and counsel you in these matters. Your doctor can provide a practical, in-depth perspective about new developments that may have been somewhat sensationalized in the media.

Scientists and researchers are expected to have high levels of integrity, ethics and accuracy in planning and conducting research. However, sometimes authors or sponsors of studies may have inappropriate influence on the planning, execution or writing up of the study. A study can end up with less accurate results or reporting. Generally, this will be picked up by their colleagues in the peer review process.

Occasionally, a concern will arise when the authors of a research report are employees of the company that manufactures the drug being tested. Many steps are taken to oversee and publish studies to ensure conflicts of interests are avoided or at least declared. Some experts feel that studies sponsored or funded by non-profit groups, universities and government research funding agencies are more reliable and have higher scientific accuracy. Others have the opinion that researchers and those involved in clinical trials are minimally influenced by who funds the study and take great care to preserve their reputations. All studies, regardless of who has planned or conducted them, should be critically analyzed and interpreted before the findings are used in making decisions about patient care.

## RESEARCH TERMINOLOGY

The following words in bold-faced type are terms that are often used in drug therapy research. We have attempted to provide a brief description of these terms so that you can better understand and interpret research findings.

The term **clinical** refers to something based on actual observation and treatment of patients as opposed to information from data or facts obtained from sources such as patient charts or other studies.

**Clinical trials** are a method of research that looks at a wide variety of healthcare topics from prevention of disease to treatment and diagnosis. They are carefully designed and carried out investigations to prove or disprove the value of a particular therapy conducted in patients who have the disease of interest. Clinical trials are done in several phases that can take several years to complete. Phases one and two are the development and testing of a new drug in humans who may not have the diseases of interest. Phase three is the clinical trial. This involves comparing the new treatment to either a placebo or to a known effective treatment already available. The effects of a treatment on a selected human population are studied to provide evidence that a medication is effective.

By designing tight **protocols** – specific steps and procedures to be carried out— the clinical trial is controlled for factors that might unnecessarily influence an outcome or results. Using these protocols, researchers choose the population or patient group and define who is allowed into the study (**inclusion criteria**) and who cannot participate (**exclusion criteria**).

Research is most applicable to individuals who are similar to the people being studied. When designing the study and looking for participants, consideration is given to such characteristics as the age, gender and lifestyle of the **study population** or **subject selection**. For example, a study population chosen from among residents of an underdeveloped country would have different lifestyles and diet than people in a developed country. Other significant factors are income level, degree of education, height, weight, family medical history or number of children. These differences could all have an effect on the outcome of the treatment being studied.

Clinical trials in osteoporosis hip fractures are generally done with post-menopausal women with low bone mineral density as this group is at greatest risk of osteoporosis and fracture. Researchers would observe this study population to see whether or not there is a difference between the fracture data from the new treatment compared with participants treated with a placebo.

When identifying a study population, consideration is given to how many people need to be recruited and included in the trial. This is known as **sample size**. Larger studies are usually better because the results are less likely due to random chance. Smaller studies may give misleading information. For example, toss a coin four times and then 100 times and compare how often heads and tails come up. The more times you toss the coin, the bigger the "sample size" of the study and the more accurate the results are in describing what is happening.

Another consideration is how the study is conducted. This can impact the strengths and weaknesses of the medical research. Ideally, the study is **randomized**, **controlled** and **double-blinded**. For quality research and reduce bias, the study population is randomly divided into people who will receive the new treatment and people who do not receive the treatment. To further limit the bias, it is important to blind the treatment, which is done by giving one pill that is the treatment and a second pill that is a placebo (sugar pill). Both pills look identical and neither the investigators nor participants (double-blind) know which is which.

## Understanding the Results

Once all the information has been gathered, it is statistically analyzed to see if the treatment truly made a difference or if the findings happened by chance. Using **statistical analysis**, researchers can identify how confident they are about the differences and the likelihood that these differences happened by pure luck or chance.

The **p value** is a statistical measure to determine if the results observed were due to chance arising from some statistical weakness. The lower the p value, the more confident the findings are real. For example, p value < 0.05 means there is a less than five in a 100 chance that something occurred by luck or chance. Therefore, 95 times out of 100, the results would be explained as the drug effect. It is generally accepted that the effect of the treatment is not due to chance if the p value is less than 0.05.

A doctor will consider the clinical importance of a treatment based on the **clinical significance** as well as the **statistical significance**. For example, a study might show that a drug reduces bone loss (statistically significant), but it does not prove that the drug reduces fractures, which would be important clinically (clinical significance) to the doctor. Another example might be a drug treatment that may increase your duration of sleep by two minutes a night, which may be statistically significant. However, the clinical significance of this is minimal in that two minutes does not mean a lot when you already sleep six hours in a night. Both results are interesting, but they are not of clinical importance to the doctor or patient.

You will also read about the **relative risk** and **absolute risk** of the results. It is important to recognize the difference between relative risk and absolute risk. For example, imagine a study that showed a new drug would reduce the risk of fracture. The study had 100 people on the new drug and 100 people not on the drug. The study found that 10 people fractured when not on the drug. However, there were still three people that fractured even though they were on the drug. The headline might read "New drug shows 70 percent reduction in fractures."

Ask yourself: Does the 70 percent mean that 70 out of 100 people on the drug did not fracture when taking the drug (relative risk) or does the 70 percent mean that of those taking the drug, seven fewer people fractured as compared to the 10 people that might have fractured if they were not on the new drug (absolute risk).

Another interesting statistic is the **number needed to treat (NNT)**. NNT is a way to express absolute risk. It is a way of looking at the outcome of how many patients you need to treat to have one success. For example, when testing a drug to see if it will decrease fracture risk, how many people will need to be treated in order to see one fracture prevented.

Doctors are often asked by insurance companies or governments for the NNT. The number needed to treat varies with the effectiveness of the treatment and the risk of the event in the group being studied. A highly effective treatment requires just a few people with severe disease to be treated to have one less fracture. However, a less effective treatment for people with severe disease may require treating many more individuals to reduce one fracture. This is an important statistic because one of the factors often taken into consideration when deciding whether or not to cover a treatment is the number needed to treat to achieve the intended result.

The next time you read or hear a headline that makes you consider changing your medication or lifestyle, don't ignore it. But don't accept it at face value either. Ask questions about the study or treatment and talk with your healthcare provider before you make a change. Be sure the change does not have unintended consequences that you do not want.

### HAVE YOU CONSIDERED PARTICIPATING IN AN OSTEOPOROSIS STUDY?

Things to ask or consider:

- *Is the study being conducted by reliable and responsible osteoporosis investigators?*

- *Has your doctor recommended this study?*

- *Will the study offer you a potential benefit that you otherwise would not receive outside of the study? For example, will you receive a treatment that is not yet available when other treatments have failed?*

- *Is the study safe for you? What are the risks involved?*

- *Will the study arm that is placebo (sugar pill) put you at risk for the duration of the study?*

- *Will you be invited to receive the active drug after the study if you were on the placebo arm of the study?*

- *Will the study require numerous and lengthy visits?*

- *Will travel expenses and parking be covered?*

- *Are you given a chance to say no to the study without your osteoporosis care being affected?*

- *Are you being aggressively recruited to a study that you are not interested in to treat your osteoporosis?*

- *Has someone reviewed the consent form with you and have you been encouraged to discuss the study with your family and your doctor?*

- *Most importantly, has the study investigator taken the time to explain options and possible side effects in detail? Is written information provided?*

## CHAPTER 12: KEY POINTS

- **Reading a headline doesn't mean you need to change your medication. Dig deeper and discuss it with your healthcare provider.**

- **Evaluate the credibility of what is being said and how it applies to you.**

- **Health choices should be based on valid evidence from scientific research. We can and will always discover more.**

- **If you read study results, be sure you understand the terminology. Ask yourself what the results mean and how they apply to you.**

- **Clinical trials and studies are conducted in a very exact manner, but there may be weaknesses in the study design or procedures.**

**PART FOUR**

# Taking Control of Your Bone Health

**Bringing It All Together**
**Living Well with Osteoporosis**
**Examples of Patients with Osteoporosis**
**Resources**
**Glossary**

## CHAPTER 13

# Bringing It All Together

Healthcare is constantly changing. The roles of doctors and other healthcare providers are shifting. Seldom does a doctor make a house call or take sole responsibility for the treatment recommended. Managing a chronic disease, such as osteoporosis, is now a collaborative effort that requires doctors, pharmacists, dietitians, physical therapists, nurses, the patient and sometimes the patient's friends or family working together. As the patient, you are a participant and the person who brings a unique knowledge to the team. You are the expert in how you behave, what you desire and what you will and will not do to reach your desired outcome.

Research shows that people do better if they participate in their own care. Those who seek information and ask questions tend to be able to maintain a better quality of life.

For example, if the doctor says the medication you need requires a needle every day, and you dislike needles and will not follow through, then discuss that with your team. You are not the first person to dislike needles. The team may have several other options or ideas on how to manage this issue. If necessary, discuss a compromise in order to meet or to come as close as possible to the desired goal. Remember, they see hundreds of people in a year where you may only have the valuable, but limited experience of one.

## MANAGING THE PREVENTION OF BONE LOSS

Become your own best advocate. Take an active role in your bone health and you will have better outcomes, be more satisfied and treatment will be more successful. A passive patient is less likely to have as positive an outcome. Be committed to gathering credible information about the disease. Talk with friends, colleagues, local and national organizations, and your doctor to find experts in bone health. Put together a patient-centered care team list of healthcare providers that you trust. Have a discussion about patient involvement with your doctor and healthcare providers. Be sure your healthcare team understands and agrees that you are responsible for and have the right to be engaged as a decision maker in your bone healthcare.

Learn to be comfortable in discussing your concerns, preferences and desires with your team. Speak up for yourself. View yourself as an expert on you – how you cope and what you value. Understand what the disease means to your independence and quality of life so you are motivated to learn all you can and implement the decisions you have made. Healthcare professionals bring expertise and clinical practice experience about bone health and diseases. They offer education, support and assistance with problem solving. They provide options for discussion, including risks and benefits of those options. Follow through on the decisions that you and your team have agreed upon. Your objective as a team member is to work with the team to minimize bone loss as you age, to maintain and build bone (if possible), to prevent fractures and improve your quality of life.

To succeed in this approach, you, as your own advocate, will want to adapt your positive, assertive, attitudes and behaviors to reflect your desire to be informed, involved and responsible for the decisions about your bone health and treatment. As a team member, you bring expertise from your life experiences that will affect the treatments that are suggested for you.

## Develop a Management Plan

With a little guidance, education and possibly a few lifestyle changes, your bones may remain healthy for years. As your own advocate, be prepared when you meet with anyone on the team. You can facilitate this by developing a bone health care plan and file.

- *Start by writing down your assessment results from the osteoporosis and fracture risk assessments addressed in Chapter 8. This will give you a general assessment of your bone health status.*

- *Second, write down your calcium and vitamin D intake as outlined in Chapter 5. If you need assistance, contact a registered dietitian. Adjust your dietary intake as necessary.*

- *Assess how active you are. Write down your daily exercise routine and if it includes weight-bearing, muscle strengthening and balance exercises as well as other activities. Review Chapter 7. If you need help, contact a physical therapist or trainer specializing in bone health programs. Develop and commit to an exercise routine that will improve your bone health.*

- *Review Chapter 8: Clinical Evaluation to Assess Bone Health and Fracture Risk. Write down any questions that come to mind. Be informed about assessment options when you next talk with your doctor. If you have any major risk factors or a few minor risk factors, consider having a bone mineral density test. Studies show that people tend to take better care of their bones if a review of their bone density shows they are at risk.*

- *Finally, use one of the fracture risk assessment tools in Chapter 9 to establish your own 10-year fracture risk. If you show low or high bone density, follow up with your doctor for a thorough clinical assessment of your bone health. If your bone density is normal, then follow up with your doctor in a year provided nothing else changes. See the Bone Health Care Plan on page 251 for an overview of assessment.*

If you are diagnosed with low bone density, discuss your assessment and ask your doctor for his or her opinion on the value of a more detailed bone and fracture risk assessment. Your doctor can put things into perspective based on your medical history. By being informed about bone loss prevention and treatments, you will be able to communicate your concerns clearly. Be aware that low bone density alone becomes important as you age. If you are under 60, you are not facing an emergency, but you should start thinking ahead.

As you gather information and meet with healthcare professionals, share your values and beliefs about medical treatments and taking medications. Be open to listening to their expertise. Be sure you understand the risks and benefits should you choose not to exercise, not to change your diet or not to take the medication at this time.

If you are concerned and motivated, work with your team and management plan to change some of your behaviors to begin to improve your bone health through adequate calcium and vitamin D intake, appropriate exercises and a healthier lifestyle.

If you are diagnosed with osteoporosis, you will become more involved with your healthcare team as you learn to manage living with this chronic disease. Communication and education are integral to preventing future fractures. Follow the patient-centered care approach discussed earlier. Use the education, support and encouragement provided by your healthcare team to deal with challenging situations that arise as you manage your disease.

## MANAGING YOUR OSTEOPOROSIS

Knowledge and understanding are essential to so many things in our lives, especially our health and wellness. The more we know about a subject, the more confident we are and likely to be involved, participate and prevent further disease. We enjoy a sense of pride, accomplishment, achievement and self-respect as we learn new things. We feel our accomplishment as we step into a partnership

Manage your osteoporosis through a multidiscipline integrated healthcare team approach. You are a part of that team. Do not hesitate to ask questions.

with others in the management of our care. We are able to make informed choices about our care, treatments and quality of life. Once we accept that osteoporosis is a part of our lives, we can begin finding better ways to live well with the disease using our bone health care plan and file. Here are some ways you can participate in managing your disease.

## Be Prepared for Your Appointments

Keep a binder, file or notebook that includes the details, dates and duration of things connected to your medical history, recent treatments and health issues, such as:

- *Symptoms and previous fractures*
- *Medications, dosages, times taken, any side effects and when they occur*
- *If or when you started medication for osteoporosis or other conditions*
- *Past health issues and when diagnosed*
- *Lifestyle choices (amount of alcohol, caffeine intake, smoking, etc.)*
- *Physical activity past and present*
- *Meetings with physical therapists, nurses, pharmacists, dietitians or other healthcare providers*
- *Your family's current health and medical history*
- *Names of non-prescription medications, such as supplements, dosages and any side effects experienced*
- *Documents related to previous relevant X-rays and bone densitometry results*
- *Height at age 21 and current height*
- *General dietary calcium and vitamin D intake*
- *Questions you think of between visits*

Take this binder or file to your appointment and use it as a reference. Prepare a list of questions you have for the healthcare provider so you will remember to discuss your concerns. Keep them simple and legible. Before you leave the appointment, be sure to ask what follow-up treatment and appointments are needed.

An important source for information about you and your health status is your doctor. Make your time with your doctor count. Prioritize your questions and ask about issues that concern you the most. If you do not get all your questions asked or answered during the appointment, ask your doctor for other sources of credible information and book another appointment.

## Keep a Daily Journal or Diary

To become more aware of your disease and how it impacts your life, keep a journal or diary of each day's activities and events. Briefly make a note of how you feel, what you have done and any changes you have made. Briefly note your reactions and abilities to carry out activities in the day. Part of managing your own care is the responsibility to positively manage the challenging times or bad days.

### CHALLENGING DAYS

During challenging times or bad days, a person with a chronic disease may often go through several stages. For example, if you recently fractured a hip due to osteoporosis, you may feel stress trying to do something simple, such as putting on a sock. This stress can lead to tense muscles and anxiety about how you will accomplish this task. Your mind may wander and you may become afraid that you will sustain another fracture. Depression can add to your fatigue. So now, not only are you tired from trying to put on your sock, but your attitude has led to increased fatigue. This increased fatigue can bring on more muscle tension as you try to go on with your day. Do these stages sound familiar?

By keeping a journal, you can look back and see what events triggered your reaction. You may be able to recognize and change an event or its outcome to avoid the bad situation. Develop a "go to" list of things to help distract or interrupt these stages. Ideas for the list include reading, watching television, listening to music, crafts such as needlepoint, pain management techniques, meditation, deep breathing, a walk, a phone call or even rest and focus on happier thoughts. One section of your journal can be reserved for "the good things." These can be the simple things that, even on a bad day, you are grateful for, such as a visit or phone call from a good friend or grandchild, a pleasant meal, a gorgeous sunset or a good joke that made you laugh out loud. Try it. It may take a while to remember to look at your "go to" list during a bad day, but it may just be what you need to break the cycle.

## Appointment and Test Result File

Make a list of all your doctors and healthcare providers along with their locations, phone numbers and when you see them. After each appointment, briefly note what was discussed or learned and any changes to your treatment plan. Keep a list of tests requested and results. Ask for copies of the results or write down the results you were told.

## Information File

Set up a file to hold articles or information on good resources, exercise programs, public forums, support groups and health professionals specializing in bone health.

## Medication Calendar

Use a calendar or notebook to record the day, time and dosage of your supplements and medications, when they need to be renewed and any drug reactions you may have, either positive or negative.

Also note any changes to supplements and medications, including the brand name.

As the patient-partner of your healthcare team, you are responsible for bringing an attitude that shows your willingness to listen, learn and discuss, and your respect for the experience of the other team members. The information you keep in your files demonstrates to the other team members that you are listening and making an effort to maintain your bone health. It indicates your understanding of the team's need for accurate information and a respect for the time limited appointment.

## Taking Medication

If you decide you will benefit from medication, make sure you take it. Medications are effective in reducing fractures from osteoporosis within just 12 months. However, only one of four people who are prescribed a medication takes the medication as they should. Almost half discontinue the medication all together.

Research studies and outcomes are based on people taking the drug as prescribed. Some drugs are not effective if not taken exactly as prescribed. Talk to your pharmacist to clarify uncertainties.

The good news is that studies have shown that, over a three-year period, you can reduce your risk of a fracture by 50 percent if you make sure you take your medication correctly at least 80 percent of the time. So, if you decide it is important for your wellness and quality of life to take the medication, find a medication that matches your lifestyle and is easy for you to remember to take. Then, make sure you take the medication! If there are issues with taking medication, make sure you discuss them with your doctor and pharmacist to find another option.

## Working Together

Your doctors and healthcare providers offer you expertise, years of treating people with similar situations and an understanding of what might happen to your body given your age, gender and medical condition. The doctor and healthcare team know what you *should* do, but you know what you *will* do. Ask questions. Work with your team to discover the best outcome for you. Respect your doctor's experience and knowledge; your doctor must respect your attitude, values and beliefs.

Use your appointments to ask questions, state your understanding of an issue and then ask if your understanding of it is correct. Let your healthcare provider know if you do not understand something. If you run out of time, set up another appointment or ask for direction on where to get credible and reliable answers to your questions.

**An improvement in your health will confirm your efforts. This in turn will promote your self-esteem. An increased self-esteem adds greatly to your overall well-being.**

Ideally, your team will assess and provide current information for dietary requirements, exercise programs and medication options. Team members will share the consequences of the various alternatives with you and address concerns about psychosocial, family, community and work issues. If all these systems are not in place, be persistent and find a way to get the information and the outcome you desire.

Do not let the disease take over your life. Use the resources and support available and find a healthy way to live a balanced life while managing the disease. Focus on maintaining or improving your health. Focus on your quality of life and wellness rather than the disease.

## CHAPTER 13 KEY POINTS

- Become your own best advocate. Take an active role in your bone health. You will have better outcomes, be more satisfied and treatment will be more successful.

- Discuss your bone health and height with your doctor at each annual physical exam.

- Your role is to bring a positive attitude, behaviors that show you want to maintain or improve your bone health and to have credible information and resources.

- Develop a bone health care plan that will involve your assessment of osteoporosis and fracture risk, calcium and vitamin D levels, and activity level.

- Keep a folder or binder with appointments and decisions made, test results, questions, your medication calendar, recent articles, etc.

- If you feel you are at risk of a fracture, have a proper clinical assessment done by your doctor.

- If you are at low risk or high risk of osteoporosis, your treatment choices are clearer. If you are at moderate risk of osteoporosis, the treatment choice may be less clear.

- Communicate your thoughts and concerns to your healthcare team. Ask questions.

- Take responsibility for the decisions that are made and act accordingly.

# Living Well with Osteoporosis

Picture the last time you:

- *Walked in a crowd*
- *Hugged your children and grandchildren*
- *Carried groceries*
- *Went for a walk, hike or jog*

Did you ask yourself: "Will I break a bone?" Individuals with osteoporosis will calculate the risk and benefit of every task.

A fall or fracture may cause:

- *Fear and anxiousness that you could fall again*
- *Fear of intimacy*
- *Chronic pain from a spinal fracture or collapse*
- *Depression from the limitations of not being as mobile as you used to be*
- *Worry about a further loss of independence*
- *A diminished self-worth and self-image*
- *A change in your relationships and social roles from decreased mobility and increased pain*

Receiving a diagnosis of osteoporosis can be devastating, conjuring up thoughts of a life where you worry that every movement you make may cause bones to break.

Because osteoporosis is not always visible, other people can misunderstand your actions or choices. It can be frustrating when you want to help lift bags of groceries, suitcases or children, but you know that these activities would not be wise. Maintaining your self-esteem, independence and quality of life are important.

Healthy intimate or friendly relationships are also important as they can affect all aspects of your life. It is important to talk about what you miss, want or need from important relationships. A good relationship of any kind begins with honest communication.

In this chapter we offer some suggestions for living well with osteoporosis – to help you cope with daily movements and activities, and manage pain. More information on these issues as well as on chronic pain and relationships can be found on our website osteoporosisbook.com

## DAILY MOVEMENT AND ACTIVITIES

### Lying Down on a Bed

- *Sit on the side of the bed.*

- *Use your arms to lower yourself down onto your side as you bring your legs on the bed.*

- *If you wish, put a pillow between your knees to relieve the pressure from your back*

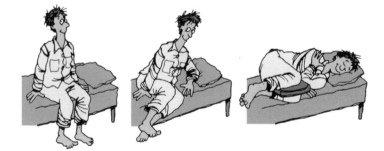

## Sitting Up on a Bed

- *When changing from a lying position to sitting, roll onto your side.*

- *Use both hands to push yourself up into a sitting position (without bending forward) as you move your legs off the bed and your feet move toward the floor.*

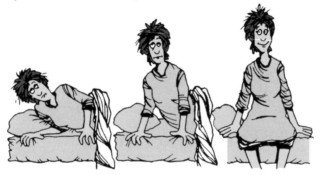

## Getting Up from a Bed

- *Roll onto your side so that you are facing the side of the bed. Keep your back straight.*

- *Sit for a few moments to feel balanced and oriented.*

- *You may find it helpful to adjust the height of the bed so your knees are at a 90 degree angle or greater. A greater angle will be even easier for standing to get out of bed.*

## Standing

- *Keep shoulders down and back, chin in and tummy in to support a natural arch in your lower back.*

- *If you must stand in one place for several minutes, such as standing at a sink, relieve the pressure on your back by placing one foot on a stool, keeping your tummy tucked in and pelvis square. Remember to switch to the other foot periodically.*

## Bending

- *Bend from your knees. Maintain a flat upper back and natural low back curve (see Posture in Chapter 6).*

- *Do not bend and twist. With movements such as those you use for vacuuming, try a rhythmic side to side or forward and back motion. To do this, bend your knees, keep your shoulders back and rock from foot to foot.*

- *A cough or sneeze may result in a sudden forward bend. To protect the spine from this sudden forward bend, develop a habit of supporting your back when coughing or sneezing. Apply this support by pulling your tummy in and placing your hand against the small of your back when you are about to cough or sneeze.*

- *To change the direction you are facing, move your feet with your body. Bend your knees slightly and pivot on your toes or heels.*

- *Remember, bend at your knees, not from your back when putting groceries into or out of the basket.*

A key element to living well is social interaction. Be fitted with and learn to use mobility aids so you can go out with friends.

Walkers and canes can give you the freedom to do your own shopping or to go for a walk in the park. They will help you to maintain your strength.

## Lifting

- *Do not lift anything while you are bending forward.*

- *If you must lift something, be sure you are properly balanced. Place your feet about one foot apart.*

- *Bend at the knees with your back straight and then squat down. Hold the item you are lifting close to your body.*

- *Use your legs, not your back, to lift, straightening up gradually without jerking.*

## Carrying

- *Avoid carrying heavy packages that may cause you to strain your back or lose your balance.*

- *If you must carry something, carry it close to your body or distribute the weight between both arms and over the larger joints, such as the shoulders.*

- *Avoid obstruction of your vision when carrying large parcels or packages. A shopping basket with wheels can be helpful.*

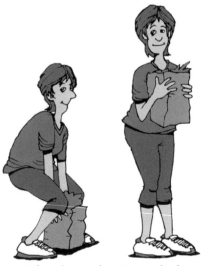

**Lift and carry close to your body**

## Back Support

- *Orthopedic back supports, such as back braces, are designed to support the lumbar spine and to assist with good posture. While providing support to the spine, the brace may also lessen movement of the back muscles. Lack of movement may help decrease the pain, but other problems may occur over time if not carefully monitored.*

- *Most doctors avoid recommending a back brace.*

- *If a brace must be used, it should be used in conjunction with an appropriate, regular and frequent exercise program to ensure that the back muscles are properly worked and strengthened.*

## Sitting in a Chair

- *Place a two to four inch rolled towel or small pillow behind your lower back to support the natural arch in your back.*

- *Use a neck rest to support the curve in your neck.*

- *If working at a desk or reading a book, prop the work up on a clipboard or against several books so that it slants toward your body. This position will allow you to maintain your correct sitting posture, and you will find that your body does not tire as quickly.*

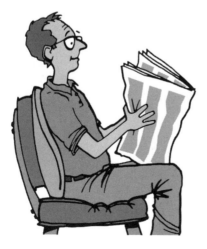

## Driving

- *If you have had a compression fracture, you may be concerned about driving a car. There is no clear answer about whether or not you should drive.*

- *Initially, personal pain and the safety of others may result in a decision to avoid driving for a while.*

- *Flexibility of the neck and shoulders are important in determining readiness to drive. As the range of motion and your strength increases, there is no medical reason why you should not drive again. A firm seat with a good back support and automatic gear shift will make the return to driving easier.*

## Gardening

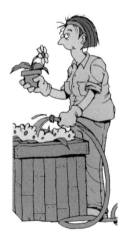

- *Use raised garden beds so you can sit or stand to garden comfortably.*

- *Use an irrigation system or a longer hose to avoid carrying water to the plants.*

- *Use a two-wheeled wheelbarrow to reduce the stress on your back.*

- *Use a pulley system to lower and raise light hanging baskets for easier care.*

- *Bend at the knees rather than the waist to pick up items.*

- *Rake leaves by using your legs to shift your weight rather than twisting your back.*

- *Wear garden gloves with rubber grips so tools are easier to control.*

- *Wear shoes with rubber or skid-resistant soles to minimize the risk of falling.*

## Walking

- *Walking has many health benefits, such as improved muscle strength, balance, circulation and even weight loss. It can be a family or social activity or a solitary meditative opportunity. Most importantly, walking is usually gentle on the body and will have an impact on your bones.*

## DAILY LIVING TASKS

### Reaching

- *Avoid reaching that requires bending and twisting.*

- *Use a "reacher" whenever possible to assist in reaching, so you avoid the flexion of leaning forward and down. Reachers can be used for many chores, such as picking up clothing.*

#### LONG HANDLES

- *Long handles are used to reduce forward bending. Examples are a long shoe horn, stocking or shirt aids, long-handled combs, gardening tools.*

- *A long-handled bath brush or double-handled scrub towel will help you reach your back.*

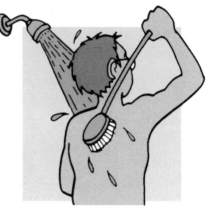

**Long Handle Bath Brush**

- *An electric broom or a long-handled dust pan will avoid the flexion of leaning forward.*

- *A hand-held shower attachment prevents unnecessary stretching.*

## Household Chores

- *Discuss household chores (washing floors, scrubbing sinks, tubs and toilets, dusting and vacuuming) with your doctor or physical therapist. Many chores are very stressful on the back.*

- *Ask your family or friends for help. If financially possible, consider having a cleaning service weekly, biweekly or monthly for a while.*

## Kitchen

- *When cooking something like a big pot of stew or soup, put the pot on the stove while empty. Add all the ingredients to the pot. Once the food is ready for serving or freezing, serve the portions directly from the pot on the stove to the dish or freezer container you intend to use. You will have a lighter, empty pot to lift and place into the sink.*

- *Use a steamer basket in your pot of water for cooking vegetables. You can lift out the vegetables without having to lift a heavy pot of water and vegetables.*

- *Use the front half of lower cupboards for your most used items. If possible, have the cupboards adjusted so that the shelves slide out. This applies to any room.*

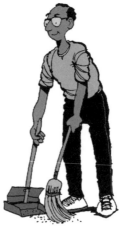

**Long Handle Dust Pan**

## Bathroom

- *Use a hand towel instead of a bath towel or bath sheet to dry yourself, as it will be lighter and easier to manage if the movement of using a bath towel causes pain.*

- *Use soap on a rope to prevent the need to bend forward in a flexed position to reach the soap.*

- *Medical supply stores have many helpful aids, such as a toilet seat lift (with handles to help you raise yourself) and bathtub seats.*

Review Fall Prevention in Chapter 10 for more safety ideas.

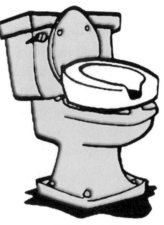

**Toilet Seat Lift**

## MANAGING PAIN

Unfortunately, pain can affect our attitude, behavior and ability to cope with any situation. Pain is a way the body lets us know that something is not right. Ideally, we should be able to recognize pain, find out why the pain is occurring, correct the cause and eliminate the pain. However, sometimes correcting the cause is not simple and different interventions may be required. Knowing when and how to use medication and non-medication techniques for pain relief can be very important to your health.

The acute pain after vertebral fracture usually resolves in about six weeks. Individuals are often left with residual chronic back pain aggravated by sitting or standing for any length of time. This is due to the change in vertebral shape that causes affected muscles in the back to cramp and spasm. A physical therapist, experienced in managing symptoms associated with vertebral compression fractures, can prescribe a daily home exercise regimen designed to stretch and strengthen these muscles and thus decrease symptoms and improve back strength.

Although many people do not like to take pain medication, some medications play a very important role in your treatment program when used properly and monitored by your doctor. Keep a diary of the time you experience pain, the duration and the severity of the pain using a scale of one to 10, where one is very mild and 10 is very severe. As you improve, you and your doctor or healthcare provider should attempt to slowly reduce your pain medication to reach the lowest dose effective for you.

Generally, pain medication is prescribed for two reasons:

- *It makes you feel more comfortable so you can rest properly. Rest allows your body to have its maximum amount of energy for repair.*

- *It decreases discomfort so that you are able to move and function as normally as possible. Movement will help to keep your muscles strong and assist your body to circulate blood, which carries healing properties to the affected area.*

Some pain management techniques do not require medications. These are important when pain medication alone is not enough or when the medication is more than you need for the amount of pain you are experiencing.

Many good resources are available on these different techniques. A few common techniques are outlined below. For more information and direction in this area, check with your doctor, healthcare provider and library or search the internet. Check with your national non-profit organizations, community centers and other reliable sources for referrals to pain or chronic pain management programs.

## Heat or Cold

Applying either heat or cold to an area causes the body to increase circulation to that area. This increased circulation may help to decrease the pain. Heat can be applied using a hot water bottle. The heat will feel warm and comfortable and cause some muscle relaxation. Other products are available that make this more convenient. One is called a "magic bag." It consists of tiny balls in a cloth bag that you heat in a microwave oven or put in the freezer.

*Learn the benefits and risks of pain. Identify which pains are a healthy warning and which pains may interfere with your recovery.*

Cold is often used if the area of the pain is hot and inflamed. Cold can be applied using a bag of frozen peas. These peas can be returned to the freezer for reuse as a cold pack, but should be clearly marked so they are not opened and eaten. Applying cold in one area may cause numbness, which may temporarily decrease the pain. Be careful not to cause frostbite. Ten minutes is generally a maximum time limit to apply cold.

## Refocusing

Refocusing requires you to turn your attention away from the pain to something else. Refocusing can be accomplished through many different methods, including:

- **Distraction**, *which involves applying your thoughts to another task as you perform an activity. A mental task, such as naming a flower or bird for every letter of the alphabet, may help when doing short term activities that you know will be painful, such as climbing stairs, vacuuming or getting out of a car. For long term distraction, you may wish to try a mentally engaging and stimulating activity such as reading a book, watching a movie or becoming engrossed in a hobby, such as stamp collecting or painting.*

- **Imagery**, *where you imagine yourself in a beautiful, scenic setting. Describe all the details to yourself with special attention to the sights, sounds, smells and textures in your picture.*

- **Self-healing**, *a method similar to imagery. Picture the injured or painful area and focus your energy on that area. Imagine a well-organized team of people carrying the pain out of your body cell by cell.*

- **Dis-association** *from the pain. Picture yourself so relaxed that you can float in the air while you leave the pain behind. Start by relaxing your fingers, arms and shoulders, then your toes, feet, legs and hips. Finally, relax your seat muscles, lower back, upper back and head.*

- **Attitude**, *which may help you refocus and control pain. For example, if you do not want to get out of bed because you are comfortable and movement will cause pain, turn your attention to something positive. The idea of a hot shower or a cup of tea may make the movement worthwhile.*

## Relaxation

Relaxation exercises may help when your muscles are tense. By relaxing your muscles, movement may become easier and pain may decrease.

It is important to become familiar with the pain management techniques that work best for you in various situations. For example, applying cold to an area may work if pain is localized. However, when you are trying to sleep, but feel as if your whole body is in pain, imagery may be the best method.

Individuals with depression often sleep poorly and have less tolerance for pain. Talk to your doctor or healthcare provider about how you are coping and the challenges you face. Discuss ways to manage and improve your quality of life while living with a chronic disease.

# CHAPTER 14 KEY POINTS

- **Maintain or regain your independence. There are several ways to make many movements easier and safer, such as using long handled reachers, proper lighting, hand rails, mobility aids, etc.**

- **Pain management, either through medication or pain management techniques, can help you feel more comfortable, rest properly and help your body repair. It also decreases discomfort so you are able to move and function, which helps to keep your muscles strong. Movement also assists your body to circulate blood which carries healing properties throughout the body.**

- **Try different pain management techniques, such as heat or cold, refocusing or relaxation and medication.**

- **Read, join support groups, volunteer, research ways to remain involved with your family, friends and community.**

# CHAPTER 15

# Examples of Patients with Osteoporosis

## Robin is still losing bone density

Robin is a 69-year-old woman with severe osteoporosis. Two years ago, she developed mid-back pain while lifting a heavy suitcase. X-rays showed a fracture of the tenth thoracic vertebra. The pain settled after three months and her doctor put her on a once a week medication. A bone density test was done at the time and repeated two years later. She was dismayed because bone density of her spine had fallen five percent while she was taking medication.

### IS THIS POSSIBLE?

It is important to make sure that Robin takes her medications correctly – first thing in the morning on an empty stomach and wait at least 30 minutes (preferably longer) before eating any food. Medications should be taken with a glass of water. Do not drink coffee or milk or take other medications with your osteoporosis medication.

### SHOULD ROBIN CONSIDER OTHER MEDICATIONS?

Other options would be to take the intravenous medication zolendronic acid (Reclast, Aclasta) by infusion once yearly or switch to denosumab (Prolia) by subcutaneous injection twice a year.

## Jill suffers from kidney stones

Jill, a 53-year-old woman, was encouraged by her older sister to have a bone density test. Jill was surprised when the results showed that a T-score of her lumbar spine at -4.2 SD. In recent years, Jill had passed some kidney stones, but had no other apparent risks for osteoporosis.

### SHOULD JILL BE CONCERNED ABOUT THE KIDNEY STONES?

Hyperparathyroidism is a condition associated with kidney stones and osteoporosis. Hyperparathyroidism is overactivity of parathyroid glands resulting in excess production of parathyroid hormone. It occurs in about one in 1,000 people. Simple blood tests, including measuring serum calcium levels and a parathyroid hormone level, will confirm the diagnosis.

Jill's blood tests confirmed she has hyperparathyroidism. Her doctor recommended that she have a simple operation to remove her parathyroid glands. Normal bone density would likely be restored over several years.

## Laura is post-menopausal and wonders if she needs medication

Laura, a 57-year-old woman, asked her doctor for a follow-up bone density test. The test showed Laura had osteoporosis with a T-score of -2.5 SD. Laura thought she should go on medications for osteoporosis.

### DOES LAURA NEED TO BE TREATED WITH MEDICATIONS?

Probably not right away. Laura has no other risk factors for osteoporosis, so her risks for a fracture are relatively low. She needs to maintain a healthy lifestyle. She should have good calcium intake (1,200mg per day), take vitamin D (2,000IU per day) and do regular weight-bearing exercises (over three times a week). Her risk profile should be reviewed periodically as she gets older. Laura should do her FRAX assessment to determine her risk of fracture over the next 10 years.

## Joe recently fractured his hip

Joe is a 73-year-old man who could hardly believe it when his doctor told him he had osteoporosis. Joe always thought of osteoporosis as a "woman's disease." Recently, Joe fell taking the garbage out and fractured his hip. A bone density test showed his

T-score to be -2.7 SD. The doctor said that his lifestyle that included smoking (he quit six months earlier) and consuming two to three beers a day might have contributed to his poor bone health.

### SHOULD JOE BE ON MEDICATIONS?

Joe needs to keep active and probably limit his beer consumption to one to two a day (recent medical evidence supports that some beer may actually be beneficial, but not in excess). Joe says he does not want to take medications. However, his doctor advises that taking medications for the next five years or so is a good idea as it will help to build up his bones.

## Walter's chest X-ray is showing vertebral fractures

Walter, a 75-year-old man, has had a number of medical problems in recent years. He thought it best to enter into a retirement home after his wife died unexpectedly. Walter's family doctor mentioned that his chest X-ray showed several small fractures in the thoracic spine that may have existed for several years. Walter was also surprised when the doctor told him that he had lost 1.5 inches (4 cm) in height over the last two years. Walter's FRAX assessment showed that he is borderline high risk (20 percent) of fracture over the next 10 years.

### SHOULD WALTER GO ON MEDICATIONS FOR OSTEOPOROSIS?

Walter's family doctor feels that the last thing Walter needs is a fractured hip, considering his tendency to fall and his heart condition. His doctor suggested that, in addition to taking calcium and vitamin D and doing regular exercises, Walter should take medication either once a week, intravenously once a year or as an injection under the skin twice a year.

## Wendy was treated for breast cancer

Wendy was treated for breast cancer in her early 50s with a mastectomy and received radiotherapy. She was told to avoid estrogen. Over the last 22 years, she has had a good exercise program and has tried to avoid taking medications. Recently, she fell and fractured her upper arm and was treated in a sling. She had a bone density test that showed she had osteoporosis in the lumbar spine and hip. Wendy did her FRAX and found that she had a moderate risk (18 percent) of osteoporotic fracture over the next 10 years.

Of all hip fractures, 70% may be the result of osteoporosis with the other 30% estimated to be from major trauma.

### SHOULD WENDY BE ON MEDICATIONS FOR OSTEOPOROSIS?

Probably. Wendy has been cancer free for more than 20 years. One of the biggest concerns for her health over the next few years would be another major osteoporotic fracture, such as a hip fracture. Estrogen would probably not be advised given her age and history of breast cancer. Options to discuss with her doctor would include selective estrogen receptor modulators (SERMs), bisphosphonates or denosumab.

## Bob broke his collar bone and is worried about osteoporosis

Bob is a 62-year-old who has completed several marathons over the last 10 years. He also enjoys cycling. Recently, he fell off his bike and broke his collar bone and a low thoracic vertebra. A bone density test showed that he had slightly lower bone density than would be expected. Bob did his bone FRAX and found that he had a low risk (eight percent) of osteoporotic fracture over the next 10 years.

### SHOULD BOB GO ON MEDICATIONS?

Probably not. Bob has had traumatic fractures from his active lifestyle. Anyone at any age might break a bone with significant traumatic force. Over time, Bob's fracture should heal and then he needs to lead a healthy lifestyle with diet and good exercise.

Bob might want to re-evaluate the type of cycling he does. He should consider not going down mountain trails with his grandson, for example.

## Mary recently fell, did not break a bone, but was diagnosed with osteoporosis

Mary, a very active 75-year-old, walks her daughter's dog during the day when her daughter is working. Recently, her daughter got another young, big dog that is not well trained. Mary was not surprised when she was pulled over by the dog at the dog park. Fortunately, she landed in a bush, cushioning her fall, and she received only some scrapes, but no broken bones. Her doctor told her that her bones were thin and might break.

### WHAT SHOULD MARY DO?

Mary might have osteoporosis and will find out when her bone density is done next month. In the meantime, she has spoken with her daughter about the risk of another fall and what it could mean if she fractures a bone. Mary plans to keep walking, but not with her daughter's untrained dog. Instead, she has found a new walking partner.

Mary's bone density test reveals that she has osteoporosis. Two fractures of the spine also showed up on the radiograph (X-ray) of the bone density test. Mary agrees to go on a medication for osteoporosis, which she later learns that her new walking partner has been taking for the last two years.

## Violet has malabsorption issues due to celiac disease

Celiac disease is a common medical condition caused by an allergy or intolerance to gluten, which is a protein in wheat and other grains. Common symptoms of celiac disease include weight loss and diarrhea. Malabsorption of important nutrients, such as calcium and iron, may be the only presenting features. The diagnosis is easily made by a blood test in symptomatic patients. Only occasionally will a small bowel biopsy through an upper endoscopy or scope (a tube with a camera that enters the stomach through the mouth) be required. If calcium and vitamin D are malabsorbed, then bone loss resulting in fractures may occur.

The preferred treatment is to avoid gluten through a strict diet that does not include wheat, oat, rye and other grains. It is important to get extra calcium and vitamin D.

### SHOULD VIOLET BE CONCERNED ABOUT OSTEOPOROSIS?

Violet's FRAX assessment shows that she is at borderline normal risk (nine percent) of osteoporotic fracture over the next 10 years. If her next assessment shows significant bone loss, then she might consider taking a medication.

## Bill is on treatment and still losing bone

Bill follows a treatment of medication, calcium and vitamin D, and has made lifestyle changes as suggested by his doctor, but he is still losing bone. Bill has been good at following the directions and taking his osteoporosis medication.

### WHAT SHOULD BILL DO?

Bill might need to be seen by a specialist to make sure that all secondary causes of osteoporosis are ruled out. This can usually be done through routine blood tests. Occasionally, a bone biopsy or bone marrow biopsy might be suggested.

It is important to know that, depending on equipment and the positioning, results of bone density tests can vary by up to several percent. Bill's doctor may want to consult with a radiologist or other specialist to confirm that Bill's test results were read correctly.

Bone density can change dramatically due to significant weight loss. Charts that attempt to show corrections in bone density measurements associated with changes in body weight are not always accurate for some individuals. Other variables often come into play.

If it is confirmed that Bill's bone density has fallen while on treatment, then consideration should be given to switching to a different medication, such as bisphosphonate by intravenous injection, denosumab or parathyroid hormone. He should continue with his lifestyle change that includes taking calcium and vitamin D and exercising regularly.

## Betty has been on prednisone for several years

Betty, 55, has had rheumatoid arthritis for seven years. The disease is moderately active and she had been on low-dose prednisone for many years to control her symptoms. Since her doctor put her on a biologic medication for rheumatoid arthritis, which she regularly self-injects, Betty has experienced dramatic improvement and has stopped taking the prednisone.

### SHOULD BETTY GO ON A MEDICATION FOR OSTEOPOROSIS?

Possibly. Rheumatoid arthritis is commonly associated with bone loss because of active inflammation, decreased physical activity and medications such as prednisone. As Betty's rheumatoid arthritis has been active for seven years and she had been taking prednisone for a few years, she has two important risk factors for osteoporotic fractures. To determine if she is prone for fracture, Betty did a 10-year risk assessment using FRAX. It turns out that her bone density T-score of the hip is quite low, but her mother had a hip fracture, so her 10-year risk of a major osteoporotic fracture is high. Betty should be reminded to get good calcium and vitamin D supplements if her diet is not good. She is considering a medication her doctor recommended.

## Margaret is going through menopause and worries about osteoporosis

Margaret is a 50-year-old who has recent onset of hot flashes at night resulting in poor sleep. Her periods have been irregular the last three months. Recently, an elderly aunt of Margaret's broke a hip.

### SHOULD MARGARET GO ON MEDICATION FOR OSTEOPOROSIS?

Peri-menopause can be very stressful and Margaret needs to make the right choice in regard to her bone health. She sees this as an opportune time to do a bone density test and a risk assessment calculation. Calculation of a 10-year risk assessment with FRAX can be very reassuring.

Margaret has no significant risk for osteoporosis and her calculated risk of a fracture over the next 10 years is low (seven percent). She is considering going on a low dose of estrogen for a short period to help her transition through menopause. She knows she probably won't need to take the estrogen for long. Margaret has read about osteoporosis and plans to have good calcium and vitamin D supplementation and to increase her regular exercise to improve her general health.

## James has malabsorption issues and a compression fracture

James, 35, has had Crohn's disease since he was in his early 20s. He has had several bowel surgeries and also has received high doses of prednisone for months at a time.

### SHOULD JAMES BE ASSESSED AND STARTED ON TREATMENT FOR OSTEOPOROSIS?

Patients with Crohn's disease have a high incidence of osteoporosis because of poor diet, malabsorption of nutrients, secondary hyperparathyroidism (the parathyroid glands working overtime because of low serum calcium) and the frequent use of prednisone.

James should have blood tests to rule out malabsorption and probably a bone density test to help estimate risk of future fracture. A bone density test is less useful in younger people for a variety of reasons, but it may give a good baseline.

James' doctor emphasizes that James should maintain a good diet with calcium and vitamin D supplementation. They will try not to use prednisone. Other medications can be effective and will be considered if osteoporosis is of concern. James might be able to avoid medication if he is able to maintain a healthy lifestyle.

Unfortunately, James now has acute back pain as a result of lifting his young nephew. An X-ray showed a compression fracture of a low thoracic vertebra. James' doctor recommended that he go on a medication to avoid further fractures.

## Leslie is on a bisphosphonate and needs major dental work

Leslie is a 60-year-old woman who has been on weekly bisphosphonates for five years to treat osteoporosis. Her dentist has suggested that she have a number of implants, but he is reluctant to do any dental work as she is on medications for osteoporosis that might be associated with a jaw problem.

### SHOULD LESLIE BE CONCERNED?

Osteonecrosis of the jaw is a rare condition in people being treated with bisphosphonates for osteoporosis. It has also been reported in people not on bisphosphonates.

Osteonecrosis of the jaw presents as an area of exposed bone inside the mouth. In individuals who develop osteonecrosis of the jaw, it has been observed that 50 percent of these people have had recent dental procedures. It has been described occasionally in patients with breast, prostate or myeloma cancer who have been on monthly intravenous bisphosphonates for a year. A study of more than 7,000 post-menopausal women showed the incidence of osteonecrosis of the jaw was the same whether a woman received intravenous bisphosphonates or not. One patient in each group was equally likely to develop osteonecrosis of the jaw.

It is reasonable for Leslie to stop the bisphosphonates for one or two months and then have the dental procedure. She might even discuss with her doctor coming off bisphosphonates for a longer drug holiday.

## Brittany is suffering from anorexia nervosa

The school nurse has been counseling a 16-year-old Brittany about anorexia nervosa. She has suggested to Brittany and her parents that osteoporosis may be of concern. Anorexia nervosa is a significant medical problem that may be unrecognized in early stages. Presenting features are weight loss that occurs because of wrong assessment of self-body image resulting in an eating disorder or over exercising. Amenorrhea will often be associated with low estrogen levels from lack of ovulation. Bone loss results from nutritional malabsorption and hormonal imbalance.

## What therapy should Brittany receive?

Therapy can be a challenge. Counseling is often prolonged and may require inpatient hospital admission to address nutritional and psychological factors. Bone loss is often unrecognized and measurement of bone density may not be useful as there is so much variability. It is important to address the individual as a whole being and teach her about the importance of balanced lifestyle choices. Good calcium and vitamin D intake should be encouraged in addition to general dietary advice. Cyclic progesterone or an estrogen birth control pill might be considered. Generally, medications for osteoporosis should be avoided unless there is profound bone loss resulting in significant fractures.

# Resources

**Visit us online at osteoporosisbook.com**

The organizations listed on these pages can provide you with additional information about osteoporosis and bone health. Most can be easily found through a search of the internet or by going to osteoporosisbook.com where you will find useful up-to-date web links to the various organizations listed here.

## ILLNESS AND PREVENTION

### Centers for Disease Control and Prevention (USA)

1600 Clifton Rd.
Atlanta, GA 30333
1-800-232-4636
cdc.gov

### Institute for Safe Medication Practices

200 Lakeside Drive, Suite 200
Horsham, PA 19044-2321
(215) 947-7797
consumermedsafety.org

### National Institute of Arthritis and Musculoskeletal and Skin Diseases (NIAMS)

1 AMS Circle
Bethesda, MD 20892-3675
(301) 495-4484
niams.nih.gov

# Public Health Agency of Canada

130 Colonnade Road
A.L. 6501H
Ottawa, ON K1A 0K9
(416) 973-0003
publichealth.gc.ca

## OSTEOPOROSIS

## Foundation for Osteoporosis Research and Education (FORE)

1814 Franklin Street, Suite 620
Oakland, CA 94612
(510) 832-2663
fore.org

## National Osteoporosis Foundation

1150 17th Street NW, Suite 850
Washington, DC 20036
(202) 223-2226 or 1-800-231-4222
nof.org

## Canadian Osteoporosis Patient Network (COPN)

(Patient arm of Osteoporosis Canada)
1-800-463-6842
osteoporosis.ca

## Osteoporosis Canada

1090 Don Mills Rd, Suite 301
Toronto, ON M3C 3R6
(416) 696-2663 or 1-800-463-6842 (English)
osteoporosis.ca

## International Osteoporosis Foundation

9, rue Juste-Olivier
CH-1260 Nyon, Switzerland
+41 22 994 0100
osteofound.org

## MENOPAUSE

## The North American Menopause Society

PO Box 94527
Cleveland, OH 44101-4527
(440) 442-7550 or 1-800-774-5342
menopause.org

## The Society of Obstetricians and Gynaecologists of Canada

780 Echo Drive
Ottawa, ON K1S 5R7
(613) 730-4192 or 1-800-561-2416
menopauseandu.ca
sogc.org

## RESEARCH

## National Center for Complimentary and Alternative Medicine

P.O. Box 7923
Gaithersburg, MD 20898
1-888-644-6226
nccam.nih.gov

## National Institutes of Health

9000 Rockville Pike
Bethesda, MD 20892
(301) 496-4000
nih.gov

## National Institute on Aging

Building 31, Room 5C27
31 Center Drive, MSC 2292
Bethesda, MD 20892
(301) 496-1752  or 1-800-222-4225
nia.nih.gov

## The Women's Health Initiative

nhlbi.nih.gov/whi/

## NUTRITION

## American Dietetic Association

120 South Riverside Plaza, Suite 2000
Chicago, Il 60606-6995
(312) 899-0040 or 1-800-877-1600
eatright.org

## Office of Dietary Supplements

National Institutes of Health
6100 Executive Blvd., Room 3B01, MSC 7517
Bethesda, MD 20892-7517
(301) 435-2920
ods.od.nih.gov

## US Department of Agriculture, Center for Nutrition Policy and Promotion

3101 Park Center Drive, Rm. 1034
Alexandria, VA 22302-1594
My Pyramid Food Guidance System: 1-888-779-7264
mypyramid.gov

## Dietitians of Canada – Find a Dietitian

480 University Avenue, Suite 604
Toronto, ON M5G 1V2
(416) 596-0857
Find a dietitian: 1-888-901-7776
dietitians.ca/find

## Health Canada

Address Locator 0900C2
Ottawa, ON K1A 0K9
866-225-0709
hc-sc.gc.ca

## PROFESSIONAL

## American Medical Association

515 N. State Street
Chicago, IL 60654
1-800-621-8335
ama-assn.org

## American Pharmacists Association

2215 Constitution Avenue NW
Washington, DC 20037
(202) 628-4419 or 1-800-237-2742
pharmacist.com

## Canadian Medical Association

1867 Alta Vista Drive
Ottawa, ON K1G 5W8
cma.ca

## Canadian Pharmacists Association

1785 Alta Vista Drive
Ottawa, ON K1G 3Y6
(613) 523-7877 or 1-800-917-9489
pharmacists.ca

## JOURNAL DATABASES

## PUBMED

Comprises over 20 million citations for biomedical literature from
MEDLINE, life science journals, and online books.
ncbi.nlm.nih.gov/entrez/query.fcgi

## Cochrane Consumer Network

Online collection of databases that contain different types of
independent evidence to inform healthcare decision making.
thecochranelibrary.com

# CHAPTER 17

# Glossary

**Amenorrhea** – the absence of menstruation.

**Anabolic** – processes, usually using drugs, that cause bone tissue to build. This may be done by affecting the osteoblast cells and improving bone formation.

**Anabolic Steroids** – synthetically produced hormones that stimulate tissue growth.

**Androgen** – a substance, such as testosterone, that produces or stimulates the development of male characteristics, such as the hormone testosterone.

**Anorexia Nervosa** – eating disorder characterized by a fear of becoming obese. It can lead to osteoporosis.

**Bisphosphonates** – group of drugs used in the treatment of osteoporosis.

**Body Mass Index (BMI)** – method for assessing body weight in relation to health for most adults. To calculate your BMI, divide your metric weight by your metric height squared. A BMI of 18.5-24.9 is considered healthy for most adults.

**Bone Density** – the amount of calcium projected per square centimeter of bone.

**Bone Matrix** – intracellular (between the cells) substance from which bone is made or develops. It contributes to bone strength.

**Bone Mineralization** – final stage of bone development that hardens or stiffens bone. Bone matrix produced by osteoblasts mineralizes by the deposits of calcium apatite. The result is new bone.

**Bone Mineral Density** – average mineral concentration of a section of bone. Synonymous with bone density.

**Bone Remodeling** – process of bone resorption and formation, which is responsible for renewal of bone.

**Calcitonin** – hormone produced by the thyroid gland. Calcitonin helps save calcium in the bone. It protects the bone from loss and can be a strong analgesic or pain reliever.

**Calcitriol** – active hormone form of vitamin D that: promotes the absorption of calcium and phosphorus in the intestines; decreases calcium excretion by the kidneys; and acts along with the parathyroid hormone to maintain bone balance (homeostasis).

**Calcium** – metallic element found in most living tissues. It is required for bone formation and mineralization, muscle contraction, blood coagulation and the transmission of nerve impulses.

**CAROC** – Canadian Association of Radiologist and Osteoporosis Canada.

**Cortical Bone** – compact dense bone that forms the outer shell of all bones.

**Cortisol (cortisone, prednisone)** – hormone secreted by the adrenal glands to regulate the metabolism of fats, carbohydrates and proteins. It also acts as an anti-inflammatory agent.

**Dual-Energy X-Ray Absorptiometry (DXA)** – method used to measure the amount of bone, usually in the lumbar spine and hip. It is usually done by a machine called a densitometer.

**Estrogens** – hormones produced by the female sex glands. They are responsible for the development of sexual characteristics in women.

**Estrogen Therapy** – treatment used to correct a deficiency of estrogen, such as after menopause or after the surgical removal of ovaries.

**Fat-Soluble Vitamins** – able to dissolve in fat and stored in the body tissues.

**Fiber** – nutrient found in bran, brown rice, fruit, vegetables and some dairy products. The importance of fibre in the diet cannot be overemphasized.

**Flexion** – the act of bending forward.

**Fluoride** – chemical element that promotes the formation of bone mass. It is required by the body in small quantities for bone health. Excessive amounts lead to poor bone quality.

**Genetics** – refers to the number of body traits, such as eye and hair color, height and some diseases, that occur as a result of DNA passed on to you from your parents.

**Fragility Fracture** – occurs spontaneously, such as a fall from a standing height or less, or from a minor injury that otherwise should not fracture normal bone.

**Get Up and Go Test** – tests for mobility. Sit back in a chair with arm rests. On the word "go" stand up, using usual walking aids if needed, walk three meters in a straight line, turn, walk back to a chair and sit down. Observe for balance, foot placement, sway and gait or stride length. Less than 10 seconds is normal. Over 20 seconds is an indicator of possible higher risk of poor functional independence and higher risk of falls.

**Height Loss** – a natural occurrence as we age. A loss of 2.5 inches (6 cm) or greater compared to your historical height loss (the amount of height you have lost since your tallest measurement), or a one inch (2.5 cm) loss over three years, called prospective height loss, may be cause for concern. To accurately measure your height, first measure your height, then step away and go back and repeat the measurement twice more (see Height Measurement Tools and Techniques). These two measurements should be the same.

**Height Measurement Tools and Techniques** – to measure your height, use a wall-mounted device in which the horizontal arm of the device is placed atop your head (compressing the hair as much as possible) and affixed to the wall at a 90 degree angle. Repeat three times and use the average to determine your height. Specialized devices to measure height are called stadiometers. Also, Rib-to-Iliac Crest (hip bone) and Wall-to-Occiput and are described below.

**Hormone Therapy (HT)** – treatment used to correct a deficiency of the hormones estrogen, progesterone or testosterone.

**Hypogonadism** – condition in which the body does not produce enough sex hormone, generally estrogen in women and testosterone in men.

**Hysterectomy** – surgical removal of the female uterus.

**International Units (IU)** – measure a drug's potency, not its mass or weight.

**Kyphosis** – outward curvature of the upper spine caused by the collapse of the vertebrae.

**Lactase** – intestinal enzyme that breaks down the milk sugar, lactose.

**Lactose** – a natural sugar found in milk and milk products.

**Lactose Intolerance** – occurs when the body cannot produce enough lactase to break down the lactose, resulting in abdominal or digestive tract symptoms.

**Lordosis** – inward curvature of the lower spine.

**Low-Trauma Fracture** – low impact fracture or broken bone that occurs from a fall from a standing height or less.

**Mechanism of Action** – the means or way a drug exerts an effect on tissue or cells.

**Menopause** – the moment a women has no menstrual period after 12 consecutive months.

**Metabolism** – process whereby the body converts food into living tissue and energy.

**Milligram (mg)** – a unit of weight equal to one thousandth of a gram.

**Mineralization** – depositing of minerals in tissues.

**Multidiscipline** – several healthcare fields or disciplines (physician, nurse, pharmacist) working in collaboration to care for the patient.

**National Health and Nutrition Examination Surveys (NHANES)** – a research program of the National Center for Health Statistics designed to assess the health and nutritional status of adults and children in the United States.

**Non-Vertebral Fracture** – fractures other than those of the spine (back).

**Non-Weight-Bearing Exercises** – non-impact exercises, such as swimming.

**Nutrients** – foods that promote life by providing nourishment for growth, repair and metabolism of body tissue.

**Occiput-to-Wall** – an indicator of spinal or vertebral collapse. A Wall-to-head (occiput) measurement will help keep track of your posture. The occiput is the point on the back of your head which is the biggest protuberance. If you stand with your heels backed-up against the wall, you should be able to touch the wall with the occiput or 'protuberance' of your head when looking straightforward. If the distance between the wall and your occiput is greater than 2.5 inches (6 cm) you may have a thoracic Kyphosis (hump), which may indicate you have vertebral fractures.

**Oophorectomy** – surgical removal of the ovaries causing surgical menopause.

**Osteoarthritis** – a type of arthritis with progressive cartilage deterioration in synovial joints and vertebrae. Different than rheumatoid arthritis.

**Osteoblasts** – cells that form bone by laying down a matrix that mineralizes.

**Osteoclasts** – cells involved with the resorption (removal) of bone.

**Osteocytes** – bone-forming cells entrapped within the bone matrix that help maintain bone as a living tissue.

**Osteopenia** – occurs when bone mineral density is lower than normal, but not low enough to be considered osteoporosis. Some experts feel this may be a pre-cursor to osteoporosis.

**Osteoporotic Vertebral (spinal) Fractures (OVF)** – a fracture in the spine where bone loss in the spine has caused the vertebrae to become weak and porous to the point the vertebrae eventually collapses or breaks.

**Osteoprotegerin (OPG)** – part of the body's natural bone tissue defense. It is a protein that blocks RANKL from stimulating bone resorption.

**Oxalates** – compounds found in foods, such as beet greens, rhubarb, sorrel, spinach, summer squash, chocolate, cocoa and peanuts, that can interfere with the absorption of calcium.

**Parathyroid Hormone** – secreted by the parathyroid gland. It promotes bone resorption (removal).

**Peak Bone Mass** – the point at which your bone building and removal are equal and you have reached your maximum bone density and strength.

**Phosphorus** – non-metallic element present in all living tissue and is involved in most metabolic processes. Phosphorus and calcium are components of bone.

**Phytates** – phosphorus-containing compounds found in raw, unprocessed foods, such as legumes or outer husks of cereals, bran and oatmeal. They can interfere with the absorption of calcium.

**Placebo** – often called a sugar pill, it is an inactive substance or treatment that looks identical to the treatment being tested.

**Plain X-ray** – image taken on a focal plane to determine if a fracture of the spine has occurred. It is usually the first test done when a patient has back pain. Thirty to 50 percent of bone must be lost before this method can detect bone loss.

**Progestin** – hormone that prepares the lining of the uterus for implantation of a fertilized ovum. Synonymous with progesterone.

**Progesterone** – female hormone produced by the ovaries during the second half of the menstrual cycle.

**Progestogen** – any natural or synthetic hormonal substance that produces effects similar to those produced by progesterone.

**Quantitative Computed Tomography (QCT Scan)** – method for measuring bone density that allows direct measurement of a particular area of bone found in the spine. It does not provide T-score compatible with the WHO classification of osteoporosis.

**RANK (Receptor Activator for Nuclear Factor kB)** – protein receptor that controls the maturation of the osteoclast cells it is connected to. When this receptor is activated by RANKL, it stimulates the osteoclast to activate and break down bone.

**RANKL (Receptor Activator for Nuclear Factor kB Ligand)** – naturally-occurring protein in the body that is released by osteoblast cells and acts as the major signal to promote bone removal or resorption.

**Resorption** – removal of bone by osteoclasts.

**Retinol Equivalent** – unit for measuring the amount of retinol derived from vitamin A. One retinol equivalent equals one microgram ($\mu$g) of retinol or six micrograms of beta-carotene.

**Rib-to-Iliac Crest (hip bone)** – an indicator of spinal or vertebral collapse. As the spine collapses, the separation between the ribs and iliac crest decreases. To measure this separation, stand and place your hand on your waist, in between your hip bone and your last rib. If the separation is less than two of your fingers, you may have vertebral fractures.

**Rheumatoid Arthritis** – a chronic inflammatory disease mainly of the joints. Inflammation in other body organs and tissues can also occur. Joints are swollen, tender, warm and stiff and have limited movement.

**Sclerostin** – protein secreted by osteocyte cells, which inhibit bone formation.

**Senile Osteoporosis** – sometimes used to refer to osteoporosis that is due to the loss of bone in aging.

**Selective Estrogen Receptor Modulators (SERMs)** – drugs that interact with the body's tissues affected by estrogen. Sometimes the SERM acts like estrogen (agonist) and, at other times, it has the effect of blocking estrogen (antagonist).

**Testosterone** – the principle androgen or male sex hormone produced in the gonads. It is responsible for masculine characteristics. It is also produced by the adrenal cortex of both men and women. It affects several tissues in the body.

**Testosterone Replacement Therapy** – treatment to correct a deficiency of testosterone, such as for men who are hypogonadal.

**Thrombosis** – blood clot.

**Thyroid Hormones** – secreted by the thyroid gland that regulate metabolism.

**Trabecular Bone** – spongy, porous, less dense bone.

**Trauma** – physical injury cause by an external force.

**Ultrasound (when used to look at osteoporosis)** – a procedure that bounces sound waves through the wrist or heel to measure the bone density in that area. It is used as a screening test for osteoporosis, but further research is needed to establish its reliability for other uses. The T-score derived from ultrasound machines do not fit in to the WHO classification.

**Vertebra** – the singular of vertebrae. There are seven cervical vertebrae, 12 thoracic vertebrae, five lumbar vertebrae, five sacral (fused to form one bone) vertebrae, and four coccygeal (fused to form one coccyx) vertebrae.

**Vitamin A** – fat-soluble vitamin essential for normal growth and development. It is formed within the body from the yellow pigment of plants. The daily requirement for adults is about 1,000mg. Retinol is the form of vitamin A found in mammals.

**Vitamin D** – fat-soluble vitamin provided in the diet, manufactured by the action of sunlight on skin, or taken as a supplement. It is converted in the liver and kidney to calcitriol – a hormone that helps in the absorption of calcium and phosphorus.

**Vitamin K** – fat-soluble vitamin found in most green vegetables. It plays a role in bone metabolism and blood clotting.

**Weight-Bearing Exercises** – exercises in which weight is applied directly to the bone against the force of gravity. Examples are walking, dancing or climbing stairs. Weight-bearing exercises are necessary in order to maintain healthy bones.

# BONE HEALTH CARE PLAN

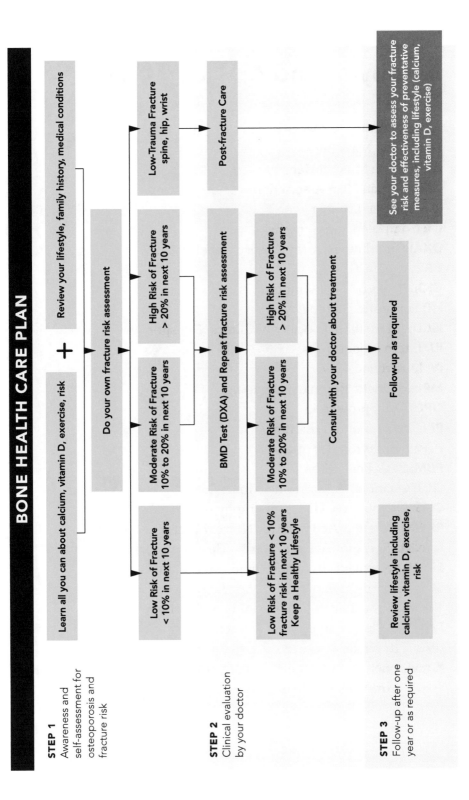

**STEP 1**
Awareness and self-assessment for osteoporosis and fracture risk

Learn all you can about calcium, vitamin D, exercise, risk

**+**

Review your lifestyle, family history, medical conditions

Do your own fracture risk assessment

Low Risk of Fracture < 10% in next 10 years

Moderate Risk of Fracture 10% to 20% in next 10 years

High Risk of Fracture > 20% in next 10 years

Low-Trauma Fracture spine, hip, wrist

**STEP 2**
Clinical evaluation by your doctor

Low Risk of Fracture < 10% fracture risk in next 10 years Keep a Healthy Lifestyle

BMD Test (DXA) and Repeat fracture risk assessment

Moderate Risk of Fracture 10% to 20% in next 10 years

High Risk of Fracture > 20% in next 10 years

Consult with your doctor about treatment

Post-fracture Care

**STEP 3**
Follow-up after one year or as required

Review lifestyle including calcium, vitamin D, exercise, risk

Follow-up as required

See your doctor to assess your fracture risk and effectiveness of preventative measures, including lifestyle (calcium, vitamin D, exercise)

# Acronyms and Abbreviations

**ADAM:** Androgen Deficiency in the Aging Male
**BMI:** Body Mass Index
**BMD:** Bone Mineral Density
**CAROC:** Canadian Association of Radiologist and Osteoporosis Canada
**CT:** Computed Tomography
**DXA:** Dual-Energy X-ray Absorptiometry
**ET:** Estrogen Therapy.
**GIO:** Glucocorticoid-Induced Osteoporosis
**HT:** Hormone Therapy
**ISCD:** International Society of Clinical Densitometry
**IU:** International Units
**IV:** Intravenous
**MRI:** Magnetic Resonance Imaging
**OPG:** Osteoprotegerin
**PPI:** Proton Pump Inhibitor
**PTH:** Parathyroid Hormone
**PBM:** Peak Bone Mass
**QCT:** Quantitative Computed Tomography
**QUS:** Quantitative Ultrasonography or Ultrasound
**RANK:** Receptor Activator for Nuclear Factor kappa-B
**RANKL:** Receptor Activator for Nuclear Factor kappa-B Ligand
**SERM:** Selective Estrogen Receptor Modulators
**SD:** Standard Deviation
**T-score:** Bone density or bone mineral density measurement
**TRT:** Testosterone Replacement Therapy
**UVB:** Ultraviolet B
**X-ray:** a method of imaging the body using small doses of radiation
**WHO:** World Health Organization

## MEDICATIONS – GENERIC NAME (BRAND NAMES)

Alendronate (Fosamax, Fosavance)
Calcitonin (Miacalcin, Fortical, Calcimar)
Etidronate (Didrocal)
Ibandronate (Boniva)
Risedronate (Actonel, Atelvia)
Raloxifene (Evista)
Denosumab (Prolia)
Teriparatide (Forteo)
Zoledronic Acid (Reclast, Aclasta, Zometa)

# Acknowledgements

The authors wish to thank those involved with the first and second edition of *The Osteoporosis Book*. The third edition is a result of all their effort and support. We are especially grateful to Dr. D. Harold Copp and Dr. Alan Tenenhouse who provided the forewords, Leslie Paris, BHE, MEd; Sandy Ganz, BPT, MEd and other health professionals who generously provided content review in their area of expertise. Thank you also to Michael Kluckner, Carole Vince, Bruce Wells, Doug Shakels, Earl Marsh, Susan Pinton, Christine Allen, Stuart Bird, Dr. Berti and everyone else who provided technical assistance, lay reviews and support and who tirelessly saw the books through to publication and marketing. A special thanks to Dr. Tim Murray for his tribute to Dr. Copp.

The third edition of *The Osteoporosis Book* was also a collaborative effort. We would like to thank Dr. Richard Bebb, endocrinologist and Dr. Tim Rowe, obstetrician and gynaecologist for their content expertise and review of all three editions covering men's and women's health issues as well as to Dr. Jonathan D. Adachi, rheumatologist for his reviews and the foreword.

We are grateful to those that participated in the third edition content reviews and updates: Dr. Brian Lentle, radiologist; Dr. Michael McClung, endocrinologist; Dr. Sonja Singh, FP; Dr. Chui Kin Yuen, Executive Director and Founder, Sigma Canadian Menopause Society; Dr. Nigel Gilchrist, consultant; Dr. David Hanley, internal medicine; Dr. Meena Sran, PT, PhD; Dr. Susie Tenenhouse; Bruce Clark, RPT; Sue North, MN; Debbie Reid, RDT; Angela Fairleigh,OT; Betsy McClung, MN; Paul Adam, MSW; Pamela Pethick, BScN; Lorraine Ellert, MA; and Tanya Long, M.Phil.

Thank you as well to those involved in the technical assistance, lay review and general support of the third edition: Bruce Wells, Raymond Mah, Gavin Chow, Barbara Kay, Susan Pinton, Liesbeth Dijkhuizen, Joyce Carlone, Kathleen Cody, Sheila Davis, Cheryl Colizza, Angela Pirozzi, Robert Bryant, Yael Greenfeld, Norm Anderson, Shereen Low, Tilman von der Linde, Raine McNeil, Denise Wade, Debbie Cheong, Rena Shields, Libby Learner, Dwayne Miner, Alan Ross and Thomas Pethick.

## ABOUT THE ILLUSTRATOR

Dave Hancock created the illustrations that appear in all three editions of *The Osteoporosis Book*. Among his other freelance endeavors, Dave illustrated *The Arthritis Exercise Book*. Dave is a high school instructor in Vancouver, Canada where he has taught art, drafting, physical education, business education, social studies and applied skills. In his spare time, Dave coaches basketball and track and field.

## FOREWORD

Jonathan D. Adachi, MD, FRCPC
Professor, Department of Medicine, McMaster University
Member, Board of Directors and Council of Scientific Advisors,
International Osteoporosis Foundation

## REVIEW

Michael McClung MD, FACP
Founding Director Oregon Osteoporosis Center
Member, Council of Scientific Advisors,
International Osteoporosis Foundation

## CONSULTANT

Brian C. Lentle, MD, FRCPC, FRCR, FACR,
Professor Emeritus, Department of Radiology,
University of British Columbia
Member of the Board, International Society of
Clinical Densitometry
Past-President of the Radiology Society of North America

# About the Authors

### Gwen Ellert, RN, BScN, MEd

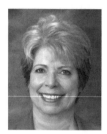

Gwen authored and published the best-selling *The Arthritis Exercise Book*. Her medical and health promotion background, in conjunction with her personal experience managing rheumatoid arthritis and risk of osteoporosis, enables her to be a strong advocate for skeletal medical issues.

### Alan Low, BSc (Pharm), PharmD, ACPR, FCSHP, CCD, RPh

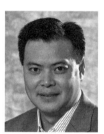

Alan is a pharmacist and a Clinical Associate Professor in the Faculty of Pharmaceutical Science at the University of British Columbia. With experience in a variety of settings, including direct patient care in hospital and clinical settings; academics; research from a hospital, university and pharmaceutical industry context; and in healthcare consulting, Alan provides a unique perspective in health education.

### John Wade, MD, FRCPC

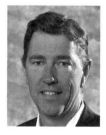

John is a rheumatologist and Clinical Associate Professor in the Department of Medicine, Division of Rheumatology at the University of British Columbia. John is active in osteoporosis research and medical and public education. He is recognized as a leading consultant at the Osteoporosis Clinic at BC Women's Health Centre in Vancouver, Canada as well as Internationally, and sits on the Professional Advisory Committee of Osteoporosis Canada, British Columbia Division.